Indian cuisine is kr and vibrant spices, ѡ٠ʳ ٠٠٠ʷ ʸ٠ʋ *can enjoy those same flavours while following a keto diet. With this comprehensive cookbook in your hands, you'll discover a treasure trove of mouth-watering Indian-style keto recipes that will transport your taste buds to a world of culinary delight.*

*"**Indian Vegetarian Keto Recipes Cookbook**" is carefully curated to bring you the best of both worlds—traditional Indian flavours and the benefits of a low-carb, high-fat lifestyle. Inside, you'll find **100 Indian Keto Vegetarian recipes** that span across all meals of the day, from breakfast to dinner and everything in between. Each recipe is thoughtfully crafted to honour the authentic Indian flavours while keeping your carb intake low.*

1 KETO PANEER BHURJI RECIPE

2 KETO VEGETABLE BIRYANI RECIPE

3 KETO PALAK PANEER RECIPE

4 KETO CAULIFLOWER UPMA RECIPE

5 KETO COCONUT CURRY RECIPE

6 KETO AVOCADO LASSI RECIPE

7 KETO STUFFED BELL PEPPERS RECIPE

8 KETO METHI THEPLA RECIPE

9 KETO MALAI KOFTA RECIPE

10 KETO EGGPLANT CURRY RECIPE

11 KETO SPINACH AND MUSHROOM SAUTÉ RECIPE

12 KETO CHIA PUDDING RECIPE

13 KETO TANDOORI CAULIFLOWER RECIPE

14 KETO MASALA CHAI RECIPE

15 KETO CABBAGE SABZI RECIPE

16 KETO COCONUT CHUTNEY RECIPE

17 KETO MATAR PANEER RECIPE

18 KETO GREEN SMOOTHIE RECIPE

19 KETO TOMATO SOUP RECIPE

20 KETO PANEER TIKKA RECIPE

21 KETO TOFU BHURJI RECIPE

22 KETO SPICED PUMPKIN SOUP RECIPE

23 KETO BAKED ZUCCHINI RECIPE

24 KETO AVOCADO SALAD RECIPE

25 KETO LEMON RICE RECIPE

26 KETO CAULIFLOWER PAKORA RECIPE

27 KETO BROCCOLI AND CHEESE SOUP RECIPE

28 KETO MUSHROOM SOUP RECIPE

29 KETO SPICY GRILLED EGGPLANT RECIPE

30 KETO MASALA ALMONDS RECIPE

31 KETO AVOCADO BOATS RECIPE

32 KETO CABBAGE SLAW RECIPE

33 KETO PALAK SOUP RECIPE

34 KETO STUFFED MUSHROOMS RECIPE

35 KETO LEMON RASAM RECIPE

36 KETO FRIED OKRA RECIPE

37 KETO CHEESE STUFFED JALAPENOS RECIPE

38 KETO BHINDI MASALA RECIPE

39 KETO TOMATO BHARTA RECIPE

40 KETO CREAMY TOMATO BASIL SOUP RECIPE

41 KETO ROASTED CAULIFLOWER RECIPE

42 KETO ROASTED BRUSSELS SPROUTS RECIPE

43 KETO PANEER MAKHANI RECIPE

44 KETO SPICY ROASTED ALMONDS RECIPE

45 KETO GREEN BEAN SALAD RECIPE

46 KETO ZUCCHINI SPAGHETTI RECIPE

47 KETO CAULIFLOWER FRIED RICE

48 KETO AVOCADO CUCUMBER SALAD

49 KETO CREAMY SPINACH SOUP

50 KETO GARLIC ROASTED BROCCOLI

51 KETO TANDOORI TOFU

52 KETO ALOO GOBI (USING CAULIFLOWER INSTEAD OF POTATOES)

53 KETO SPICED PUMPKIN SEEDS

54 KETO EGGPLANT PARMESAN

55 KETO ZUCCHINI CHIPS

56 KETO CABBAGE STIR FRY

57 KETO SPINACH AND CHEESE STUFFED MUSHROOMS

58 KETO ROASTED EGGPLANT

59 KETO CURRY ROASTED CAULIFLOWER

60 KETO ROASTED CABBAGE

61 KETO BRUSSELS SPROUTS WITH CREAMY MUSTARD SAUCE

62 KETO MUSHROOM AND SPINACH SAUTE

63 KETO ZUCCHINI NOODLES WITH CREAMY AVOCADO PESTO

64 KETO SPICY ROASTED PEANUTS

65 KETO PANEER JALFREZI

66 KETO SPICED CAULIFLOWER RICE

67 KETO BROCCOLI AND CHEESE STUFFED BELL PEPPERS

68 KETO SPICED PUMPKIN SOUP WITH COCONUT MILK

69 KETO ALMOND FLOUR ROTI

70 KETO CHILLED CUCUMBER SOUP

71 KETO BAKED CAULIFLOWER TOTS

72 KETO AVOCADO EGG SALAD

73 KETO SPINACH AND ARTICHOKE DIP

74 KETO TOMATO AND BASIL SALAD

75 KETO CABBAGE SOUP

76 KETO SPICED ROASTED CAULIFLOWER

77 KETO COCONUT AND ALMOND FLOUR FLATBREAD

78 KETO GRILLED VEGETABLE SKEWERS

79 KETO ALMOND FLOUR DOSA

80 KETO BAKED CHEESY ZUCCHINI

81 KETO SPICED ALMOND BUTTER

82 KETO MASALA ROASTED BRUSSELS SPROUTS

83 KETO PANEER AND SPINACH SOUP

84 KETO ROASTED TOMATO SOUP

85 KETO STUFFED EGGPLANT

86 KETO GRILLED EGGPLANT WITH TAHINI DRESSING

87 KETO SPINACH AND AVOCADO SALAD

88 KETO ROASTED PUMPKIN SOUP

89 KETO SPICY ROASTED CABBAGE

90 KETO GRILLED PANEER SALAD

1 Keto Paneer Bhurji Recipe

Paneer bhurji is a popular Indian dish made from crumbled paneer. In this keto version, we use healthy fats and low-carb vegetables to make it keto-friendly.

Ingredients

200 grams Paneer
2 tablespoons Olive Oil or Ghee (Clarified Butter)
1 medium Onion, finely chopped (Optional - if you want to keep carbs extra low, omit this)
1 medium Tomato, finely chopped
2 Green Chillies, finely chopped
1/2 teaspoon Turmeric Powder
1 teaspoon Cumin Seeds
Salt to taste
1/2 teaspoon Red Chilli Powder
1/2 teaspoon Garam Masala Powder
2 tablespoons Fresh Coriander (Cilantro), chopped

Instructions

- ➢ Heat the oil or ghee in a pan on medium heat.
- ➢ Add cumin seeds and let them sizzle.
- ➢ Add the chopped onions (if using) and saute until they turn translucent.
- ➢ Add the chopped tomatoes and green chillies. Cook until tomatoes are soft.
- ➢ Add turmeric powder, red chilli powder, and salt. Mix well and cook for a couple of minutes.

➤ Crumble the paneer and add it to the pan. Mix well so that the paneer is well coated with the masala.
  ➤ Cook for 5 minutes on low heat.
  ➤ Sprinkle garam masala and fresh coriander. Mix well.
  ➤ Serve hot.

Nutritional Values

Please note that these are approximate values and may vary based on exact measurements and specific ingredients used. This recipe serves 2.

Per serving:

Calories: 260
Total Fat: 20g
Saturated Fat: 8g
Total Carbohydrates: 6g (Net: 4g)
Protein: 14g

Health Benefits

High in Protein: Paneer is a good source of protein, which is beneficial for muscle growth and repair.
Healthy Fats: Ghee or olive oil provides healthy fats which are necessary for a keto diet.
Rich in Vitamins and Minerals: Tomatoes and spices like turmeric provide vitamins, minerals and antioxidants that are beneficial for overall health.

How it helps in Keto

A keto diet focuses on low carb, high fat foods. This recipe fits into a keto diet because it is high in healthy fats from the ghee or olive oil, and the paneer provides a good amount of protein. The net carbs are kept low by using a limited amount of low-carb vegetables and spices.

Best time of the day to eat

This dish is versatile and can be eaten at any time of the day. It can be a fulfilling breakfast to start the day, a lunch paired with a side of low-carb vegetables, or a light dinner. It's also a great option for a post-workout meal due to its high protein content. Remember to balance it out with other meals and snacks to keep your daily macronutrient and calorie goals.

2 Keto Vegetable Biryani Recipe

Keto Vegetable Biryani is a low-carb take on the traditional Indian dish, swapping out rice for cauliflower rice to keep it keto-friendly.

Ingredients

4 cups cauliflower rice (You can buy this pre-made or make it yourself by pulsing cauliflower florets in a food processor until they resemble rice.)
2 tablespoons ghee or coconut oil
1 onion, thinly sliced (Optional - if you want to keep carbs extra low, omit this)
2 cloves garlic, minced
1 tablespoon grated ginger
1 green chili, finely chopped
1 teaspoon cumin seeds
1 teaspoon turmeric powder
1 teaspoon coriander powder
1/2 teaspoon garam masala
1/2 teaspoon red chili powder
Salt to taste
2 cups mixed vegetables (like bell peppers, green beans, broccoli, etc.)
Fresh cilantro for garnish
A squeeze of lemon juice

Instructions

➢ Heat the ghee or coconut oil in a large pan over medium heat.

- ➤ Add the cumin seeds and let them sizzle for a few seconds.
- ➤ Add the sliced onions (if using), minced garlic, grated ginger, and green chili to the pan. Saute until the onions become translucent.
- ➤ Add the turmeric powder, coriander powder, garam masala, red chili powder, and salt to the pan. Stir to combine.
- ➤ Add the mixed vegetables to the pan and stir well to coat them with the spices. Cover the pan and let the vegetables cook until they're tender.
- ➤ Add the cauliflower rice to the pan and mix well. Cover the pan again and let everything cook together for a few minutes.
- ➤ Turn off the heat and add a squeeze of lemon juice and some fresh cilantro for garnish.
- ➤ Serve hot.

Nutritional Values

Please note that these are approximate values and can vary based on the exact measurements and specific ingredients used. This recipe serves 4.

Per serving:

Calories: 200
Total Fat: 12g
Saturated Fat: 7g
Total Carbohydrates: 17g (Net: 8g)
Protein: 4g

Health Benefits

High in Fiber: Cauliflower and other vegetables used in this recipe are high in fiber, which is beneficial for digestive health.

Low in Calories: This dish is relatively low in calories while being quite filling, making it a good choice for those looking to lose weight.

Rich in Antioxidants: Vegetables and spices used in this recipe are high in antioxidants that help to protect your cells from damage.

Good Source of Vitamins and Minerals: This dish is packed with vitamins and minerals from all the vegetables used.

How it helps in Keto

This vegetable biryani is a good fit for a keto diet because it's low in carbs and high in healthy fats from ghee or coconut oil. The cauliflower rice is a great low-carb substitute for traditional rice, keeping the net carbs in check.

Best time of the day to eat

Keto vegetable biryani is a hearty and filling dish that can be enjoyed at any time of the day. It can serve as a satisfying lunch or dinner. Remember to balance it out with other meals and snacks to meet your daily macronutrient and calorie goals.

3 Keto Palak Paneer Recipe

Palak Paneer is a classic North Indian dish. In this keto version, we'll be using generous amounts of ghee and paneer (cheese) which are high in fats and moderate in protein, ideal for keto diet.

Ingredients

200 grams Paneer
3 cups Spinach (Palak)
2 tablespoons Ghee (Clarified Butter)
1 medium Onion, finely chopped (Optional - if you want to keep carbs extra low, omit this)
1 medium Tomato, finely chopped
2 Green Chillies, finely chopped
1/2 teaspoon Turmeric Powder
1 teaspoon Cumin Seeds
Salt to taste
1/2 teaspoon Red Chilli Powder
1/2 teaspoon Garam Masala Powder
2 tablespoons Fresh Cream
1 tablespoon Ginger-Garlic Paste

Instructions

> ➤ Blanch the spinach in boiling water for 2-3 minutes. Drain and cool it down. Once cooled, blend it to make a smooth puree.
> ➤ Heat ghee in a pan, add cumin seeds and let them crackle.
> ➤ Add the chopped onions (if using) and saute until they turn golden brown.

- ➤ Add the ginger-garlic paste and saute until the raw smell goes away.
- ➤ Add chopped tomatoes and green chillies. Cook until the tomatoes turn mushy.
- ➤ Add the turmeric powder, red chilli powder, garam masala and salt. Mix well and cook for a couple of minutes.
- ➤ Add the spinach puree and cook for 5-7 minutes.
- ➤ Cube the paneer and add it to the pan. Mix well and cook for 5 minutes.
- ➤ Add fresh cream, mix well, cook for a minute and then turn off the heat.
- ➤ Serve hot with keto-friendly naan or enjoy it as a standalone dish.

Nutritional Values

Please note that these are approximate values and may vary based on exact measurements and specific ingredients used. This recipe serves 2.

Per serving:

Calories: 370
Total Fat: 28g
Saturated Fat: 16g
Total Carbohydrates: 10g (Net: 7g)
Protein: 14g

Health Benefits

High in Protein: Paneer is a good source of protein which is beneficial for muscle growth and repair.

Rich in Iron: Spinach is high in iron which can help prevent anemia.

Provides Calcium: Paneer is a great source of calcium which is necessary for strong bones and teeth.

Provides Vitamin A: Spinach is high in Vitamin A which is good for eye health.

How it helps in Keto

A keto diet focuses on low carb, high fat foods. This recipe fits into a keto diet because it's high in healthy fats from the ghee and paneer, and the paneer also provides a good amount of protein. The net carbs are kept low by using a limited amount of low-carb vegetables and spices.

Best time of the day to eat

This dish is quite versatile and can be eaten at any time of the day. It can be a fulfilling lunch or dinner. It's also a great option for a post-workout meal due to its high protein content. Remember to balance it out with other meals and snacks to keep your daily macronutrient and calorie goals.

4 Keto Cauliflower Upma Recipe

Cauliflower Upma is a great keto-friendly alternative to the traditional South Indian dish which is usually made with semolina or cream of wheat. Here, cauliflower rice is used to keep it low-carb.

Ingredients

3 cups Cauliflower Rice (You can buy this pre-made or make it yourself by pulsing cauliflower florets in a food processor until they resemble rice.)
2 tablespoons Coconut Oil or Ghee
1 teaspoon Black Mustard Seeds
1 teaspoon Urad Dal (Optional - if you want to keep carbs extra low, omit this)
1/2 teaspoon Cumin Seeds
1 Green Chilli, finely chopped
1/4 teaspoon Turmeric Powder
Salt to taste
2 tablespoons Roasted Peanuts or Cashews (Optional)
1/4 cup Green Peas (Optional - if you want to keep carbs extra low, omit this)
A handful of Fresh Coriander (Cilantro), chopped
A squeeze of Lemon Juice

Instructions

➢ Heat the coconut oil or ghee in a pan over medium heat.
➢ Add the mustard seeds, urad dal (if using), cumin seeds, and chopped green chili. Saute until the mustard seeds start to pop and the dal turns golden brown.

- ➢ Stir in the turmeric powder and salt.
- ➢ Add the cauliflower rice to the pan and mix well to combine with the spices.
- ➢ Cover the pan and let the cauliflower rice cook for 5-7 minutes until it's soft. Stir occasionally to prevent it from sticking to the bottom of the pan.
- ➢ If you're using green peas, add them to the pan and mix well. Cook for another 2-3 minutes.
- ➢ Turn off the heat and add the roasted peanuts or cashews (if using), chopped coriander, and a squeeze of lemon juice. Mix well.
- ➢ Serve hot.

Nutritional Values

Please note that these are approximate values and may vary based on exact measurements and specific ingredients used. This recipe serves 2.

Per serving:

Calories: 200
Total Fat: 16g
Saturated Fat: 10g
Total Carbohydrates: 10g (Net: 5g)
Protein: 5g

Health Benefits

Low Calorie: This dish is low in calories and can help in weight management.
Rich in Fiber: Cauliflower is high in fiber which aids digestion.

Good for Heart Health: The ghee or coconut oil used in this recipe contain healthy fats that are beneficial for heart health.

How it helps in Keto

This Cauliflower Upma is a good fit for a keto diet as it is low in carbs and high in healthy fats. Cauliflower rice is a great low-carb substitute for traditional rice or semolina, keeping the net carbs in check.

Best time of the day to eat

Cauliflower Upma is light and can be eaten at any time of the day. It is ideal for breakfast or lunch and can also serve as a quick snack in the afternoon or early evening. As always, balance it with other meals to meet your daily macronutrient and calorie goals.

5 Keto Coconut Curry Recipe

This keto coconut curry is a versatile and aromatic dish, loaded with flavorful spices and creamy coconut milk. It can be made with a variety of low-carb vegetables or even tofu for a protein boost.

Ingredients

2 tablespoons Coconut Oil or Ghee
1 medium Onion, finely chopped (Optional - if you want to keep carbs extra low, omit this)
2 cloves Garlic, minced
1 tablespoon grated Ginger
2 Green Chillies, finely chopped
1 teaspoon Turmeric Powder
1 teaspoon Cumin Powder
1 teaspoon Coriander Powder
1/2 teaspoon Cayenne Pepper (adjust to taste)
Salt to taste
1 cup Coconut Milk
2 cups mixed low-carb vegetables (like bell peppers, zucchini, spinach, etc.)
Fresh Coriander (Cilantro) for garnish

Instructions

➢ Heat the coconut oil or ghee in a pan over medium heat.
➢ Add the chopped onion (if using), minced garlic, grated ginger, and green chilies. Saute until the onions turn translucent.

- ➢ Stir in the turmeric powder, cumin powder, coriander powder, cayenne pepper, and salt.
- ➢ Add the mixed vegetables and toss to coat them in the spices.
- ➢ Pour in the coconut milk, stir well, and bring the curry to a gentle simmer. Cover the pan and let it cook for 15-20 minutes, or until the vegetables are tender.
- ➢ Check the seasoning and adjust if necessary.
- ➢ Turn off the heat and garnish with fresh cilantro.
- ➢ Serve hot. This curry can be served as a standalone dish, or it can be paired with cauliflower rice for a more filling meal.

Nutritional Values

Please note that these are approximate values and may vary based on the exact measurements and specific ingredients used. This recipe serves 2.

Per serving:

Calories: 350
Total Fat: 28g
Saturated Fat: 23g
Total Carbohydrates: 15g (Net: 10g)
Protein: 5g

Health Benefits

Rich in Healthy Fats: Coconut milk is high in healthy fats which can support weight loss, heart health, and brain function.
High in Fiber: The vegetables used in this recipe are high in fiber, promoting good digestive health.

Rich in Antioxidants: Spices like turmeric, cumin, and coriander are rich in antioxidants that protect your cells from damage.

How it helps in Keto

The keto diet focuses on high-fat, low-carb foods. This recipe fits into a keto diet as it is high in healthy fats from the coconut milk and oil, and it uses low-carb vegetables. The net carbs are kept low by using a limited amount of vegetables and spices.

Best time of the day to eat

This Keto Coconut Curry is a versatile and satisfying dish that can be enjoyed at any time of the day. It can serve as a filling lunch or dinner. Remember to balance it out with other meals and snacks to meet your daily macronutrient and calorie goals.

6 Keto Avocado Lassi Recipe

Avocado Lassi is a refreshing and creamy twist on the traditional Indian yogurt-based drink. For the keto version, we will use a low-carb sweetener instead of sugar.

Ingredients

1 ripe Avocado
1 cup plain Greek Yogurt (unsweetened)
2 tablespoons Erythritol or other keto-friendly sweetener
1/2 teaspoon Cardamom Powder
A pinch of Salt
1/2 cup Cold Water
Ice cubes
Mint leaves for garnish (optional)

Instructions

➤ Cut the avocado in half, remove the pit, and scoop out the flesh.
➤ In a blender, add the avocado, Greek yogurt, erythritol or other sweetener, cardamom powder, a pinch of salt, and cold water.
➤ Blend until smooth and creamy. Add more water if you prefer a thinner consistency.
➤ Taste and adjust the sweetness or flavoring as needed.
➤ Pour the lassi into glasses, add a few ice cubes, and garnish with mint leaves if desired.
➤ Serve chilled.

Nutritional Values

Please note that these are approximate values and may vary based on the exact measurements and specific ingredients used. This recipe serves 2.

Per serving:

Calories: 210
Total Fat: 15g
Saturated Fat: 3g
Total Carbohydrates: 12g (Net: 4g)
Protein: 8g

Health Benefits

High in Healthy Fats: Avocados are high in monounsaturated fats, which are heart-healthy and can help reduce bad cholesterol levels.
Rich in Fiber: Avocados are a good source of dietary fiber, promoting digestive health.
Good Source of Vitamins: This drink is high in vitamins such as vitamin K, vitamin E, vitamin C and B-vitamins.
Provides Probiotics: Greek yogurt is a source of probiotics, which are beneficial for gut health.

How it helps in Keto

This Avocado Lassi is keto-friendly as it is high in healthy fats from avocado, and low in carbs. Greek yogurt provides a good amount of protein, while the erythritol or other keto-friendly sweetener keeps the sugar content in check.

Best time of the day to eat

This refreshing drink can be enjoyed at any time of the day. It can serve as a great start to the morning, a cooling afternoon refreshment, or a satisfying dessert after dinner. Its high content of healthy fats can help keep you satiated and curb cravings. As always, balance it with other meals to meet your daily macronutrient and calorie goals.

7 Keto Stuffed Bell Peppers Recipe

Stuffed bell peppers make for a delicious and satisfying keto meal. This recipe uses a filling of cauliflower rice and cheese, providing a good balance of protein and healthy fats while keeping the carbs low.

Ingredients

4 Bell Peppers
2 cups Cauliflower Rice
1 cup shredded Cheese (Cheddar, Mozzarella, or a blend)
1 medium Onion, finely chopped (Optional - if you want to keep carbs extra low, omit this)
2 cloves Garlic, minced
1 tablespoon Olive Oil
Salt and Pepper to taste
1 teaspoon Paprika
1/2 teaspoon Dried Oregano

Instructions

➢ Preheat your oven to 375°F (190°C).
➢ Cut the tops off the bell peppers and remove the seeds and membranes. Place the peppers in a baking dish.
➢ Heat the olive oil in a pan over medium heat. Add the chopped onion (if using) and minced garlic, and saute until the onions are translucent.
➢ Stir in the cauliflower rice and cook for about 5 minutes, until it's slightly tender.
➢ Remove the pan from the heat and mix in the shredded cheese, salt, pepper, paprika, and dried oregano.

- ➤ Spoon the cauliflower rice and cheese mixture into the bell peppers.
- ➤ Bake for 30-35 minutes, until the peppers are tender and the filling is bubbly and lightly browned.
- ➤ Let the peppers cool for a few minutes before serving.

Nutritional Values

Please note that these are approximate values and may vary based on the exact measurements and specific ingredients used. This recipe serves 4.

Per serving:

Calories: 220
Total Fat: 14g
Saturated Fat: 6g
Total Carbohydrates: 15g (Net: 10g)
Protein: 10g

Health Benefits

High in Vitamin C: Bell peppers are very high in vitamin C, which is necessary for the growth, development, and repair of body tissues.

Rich in Antioxidants: Both bell peppers and cauliflower are rich in antioxidants, which help protect the cells in your body from damage by free radicals.

Supports Digestion: Cauliflower is high in fiber, which supports a healthy digestive system.

How it helps in Keto

Stuffed bell peppers fit well into a keto diet as they are high in healthy fats from the cheese and olive oil, and the cauliflower rice keeps the net carbs low. The bell peppers also provide a good amount of fiber, which is important on a keto diet as it can help prevent constipation.

Best time of the day to eat

These Keto Stuffed Bell Peppers are versatile and can be enjoyed at any time of the day. They make a great lunch or dinner option. Their high content of healthy fats and fiber can help keep you satiated and curb cravings. As always, balance it with other meals to meet your daily macronutrient and calorie goals.

8 Keto Methi Thepla Recipe

Methi Thepla is a traditional Indian flatbread made with fresh fenugreek leaves. This keto-friendly version uses almond flour and flaxseed meal to create a low-carb alternative.

Ingredients

1 cup Almond Flour
1/2 cup Flaxseed Meal
1 cup fresh Methi (Fenugreek) leaves, washed and finely chopped
1/2 teaspoon Turmeric Powder
1/2 teaspoon Red Chilli Powder
1/2 teaspoon Cumin Seeds
Salt to taste
2 tablespoons Olive Oil or Ghee
Water as required for kneading the dough

Instructions

➢ In a large bowl, combine the almond flour, flaxseed meal, chopped methi leaves, turmeric powder, red chilli powder, cumin seeds, and salt.
➢ Gradually add water to the mixture and knead it into a dough. The dough should be firm but pliable.
➢ Divide the dough into equal portions and roll each portion into a ball.
➢ Place one dough ball between two pieces of parchment paper or a clean, plastic-free cloth, and roll it out into a thin circle using a rolling pin.

- ➤ Heat a pan over medium heat. Place the rolled out thepla on the pan.
- ➤ Cook for about 2 minutes, or until you see bubbles appear on the surface. Flip the thepla and cook the other side for another 1-2 minutes, or until both sides are golden brown.
- ➤ Repeat with the remaining dough balls.
- ➤ Serve warm with a side of yogurt or a keto-friendly curry.

Nutritional Values

Please note that these are approximate values and may vary based on the exact measurements and specific ingredients used. This recipe serves 4.

Per serving:

Calories: 280
Total Fat: 22g
Saturated Fat: 2g
Total Carbohydrates: 11g (Net: 3g)
Protein: 11g

Health Benefits

High in Fiber: Flaxseed meal is rich in dietary fiber, which aids digestion.
Rich in Healthy Fats: Almond flour and flaxseed meal are high in healthy fats, including monounsaturated fats and omega-3 fatty acids.
Rich in Antioxidants: Methi leaves are packed with antioxidants which are beneficial for overall health.

Good Source of Protein: Both almond flour and flaxseed meal provide a good amount of protein.

How it helps in Keto

Methi Thepla fits well into a keto diet as it is low in carbs and high in healthy fats and fiber. Almond flour and flaxseed meal are both excellent low-carb alternatives to regular flour. Methi leaves add a burst of flavor without adding too many extra carbs.

Best time of the day to eat

Keto Methi Thepla can be enjoyed at any time of the day. It makes a delicious breakfast or lunch when paired with a side of yogurt or a keto-friendly curry. It can also be enjoyed as a high-fiber, high-protein snack in the afternoon. As always, balance it with other meals to meet your daily macronutrient and calorie goals.

9 Keto Malai Kofta Recipe

Malai Kofta is a classic Indian dish of dumplings in a creamy sauce. This keto version uses almond flour and paneer for the koftas, and a rich tomato-cream sauce.

Ingredients

For the Koftas:

1 cup Paneer, crumbled
1/2 cup Almond Flour
1/4 teaspoon Garam Masala
Salt to taste
2 tablespoons Fresh Cilantro, finely chopped
Oil for frying
For the Sauce:

1 tablespoon Coconut Oil or Ghee
1/2 medium Onion, finely chopped (Optional - if you want to keep carbs extra low, omit this)
2 cloves Garlic, minced
1 teaspoon grated Ginger
1/2 teaspoon Turmeric Powder
1 teaspoon Cumin Powder
1 teaspoon Coriander Powder
1 cup Tomato Puree
1 cup Heavy Cream
Salt to taste

Instructions

- ➢ Prepare the Koftas:
- ➢
- ➢ In a bowl, mix together the crumbled paneer, almond flour, garam masala, salt, and chopped cilantro until well combined.
- ➢ Form the mixture into small balls or koftas.
- ➢ Heat the oil in a pan over medium heat and fry the koftas until golden brown on all sides. Remove them from the pan and set aside on a paper towel to drain.

Prepare the Sauce:

- ➢ In the same pan, heat the coconut oil or ghee over medium heat. Add the chopped onion (if using), minced garlic, and grated ginger. Saute until the onions turn translucent.
- ➢ Stir in the turmeric powder, cumin powder, and coriander powder.
- ➢ Pour in the tomato puree and let it simmer for a few minutes.
- ➢ Add the heavy cream, stir well, and bring the sauce to a gentle simmer. Season with salt.
- ➢ Add the fried koftas to the sauce and let them simmer for a few more minutes, until heated through.

Nutritional Values

Please note that these are approximate values and may vary based on the exact measurements and specific ingredients used. This recipe serves 4.

Per serving:

Calories: 430
Total Fat: 38g
Saturated Fat: 20g
Total Carbohydrates: 10g (Net: 6g)
Protein: 14g

Health Benefits

Rich in Healthy Fats: Paneer, heavy cream, and coconut oil or ghee provide a good amount of healthy fats.

High in Protein: Paneer is a good source of protein, which is important for muscle growth and repair.

Good Source of Calcium: Paneer and heavy cream are good sources of calcium, which is essential for strong bones and teeth.

Rich in Antioxidants: Spices like turmeric, cumin, and coriander are rich in antioxidants that protect your cells from damage.

How it helps in Keto

Malai Kofta fits well into a keto diet as it is high in healthy fats and low in carbs. The use of almond flour and paneer for the koftas, and a sauce made with heavy cream, keeps the carb content low and the fat content high, in line with the macronutrient ratios recommended for a keto diet.

Best time of the day to eat

This Keto Malai Kofta makes for a rich and satisfying meal that can be enjoyed for lunch or dinner. It can be served with a side of cauliflower rice or keto naan for a complete, keto-friendly

Indian meal. As always, balance it with other meals to meet your daily macronutrient and calorie goals.

10 Keto Eggplant Curry Recipe

This recipe is for a flavorful Indian-style eggplant curry, made with spices and tomato sauce. It's a low-carb, vegetarian dish that fits well into a keto diet.

Ingredients

2 medium Eggplants
2 tablespoons Coconut Oil or Ghee
1 medium Onion, finely chopped (Optional - if you want to keep carbs extra low, omit this)
2 cloves Garlic, minced
1 tablespoon grated Ginger
1 teaspoon Turmeric Powder
1 teaspoon Cumin Powder
1 teaspoon Coriander Powder
1 cup Tomato Puree
Salt to taste
Fresh Cilantro for garnish

Instructions

➢ Cut the eggplants into cubes and set aside.
➢ Heat the coconut oil or ghee in a large pan over medium heat.
➢ Add the chopped onion (if using), minced garlic, and grated ginger. Saute until the onions turn translucent.
➢ Stir in the turmeric powder, cumin powder, and coriander powder.
➢ Add the cubed eggplants to the pan and stir until they're coated in the spice mixture.

- ➤ Pour in the tomato puree and mix well. Reduce the heat to low, cover the pan, and let the curry simmer for about 20 minutes, until the eggplant is tender.
- ➤ Season with salt and garnish with fresh cilantro before serving.

Nutritional Values

Please note that these are approximate values and may vary based on the exact measurements and specific ingredients used. This recipe serves 4.

Per serving:

Calories: 160
Total Fat: 11g
Saturated Fat: 8g
Total Carbohydrates: 16g (Net: 10g)
Protein: 3g

Health Benefits

High in Fiber: Eggplant is a good source of dietary fiber, which aids digestion and helps you feel full.

Rich in Antioxidants: Eggplant and spices like turmeric, cumin, and coriander are rich in antioxidants, which can help protect your cells from damage.

Anti-Inflammatory Properties: The curcumin in turmeric has powerful anti-inflammatory effects.

Rich in Vitamins and Minerals: Eggplant is a good source of vitamins and minerals, such as vitamin C, vitamin K, and manganese.

How it helps in Keto

Eggplant Curry can fit well into a keto diet as it is relatively low in carbs and high in fiber. The use of coconut oil or ghee adds healthy fats to the meal. As with any keto meal, portion control is key to ensure you're staying within your daily carb limit.

Best time of the day to eat

This Keto Eggplant Curry can be enjoyed as a main dish for lunch or dinner. It can be served with a side of cauliflower rice for a complete, keto-friendly Indian meal. As always, balance it with other meals to meet your daily macronutrient and calorie goals.

11 Keto Spinach and Mushroom Sauté Recipe

This simple dish of spinach and mushrooms sautéed in butter or ghee is not only easy to make but also perfectly suits the keto diet.

Ingredients

2 tablespoons of butter or ghee
2 cups of fresh spinach, washed and chopped
2 cups of mushrooms, sliced
2 cloves of garlic, minced
Salt and pepper to taste
A squeeze of fresh lemon juice (optional)
Grated Parmesan cheese for garnish (optional)

Instructions

- Heat the butter or ghee in a large skillet over medium heat.
- Add the minced garlic to the skillet and sauté until it becomes aromatic.
- Add the sliced mushrooms to the skillet and sauté until they begin to brown.
- Add the chopped spinach to the skillet. Continue to sauté until the spinach wilts.
- Season with salt and pepper. Add a squeeze of fresh lemon juice, if desired, for a bit of tang.
- Serve the spinach and mushroom sauté hot, garnished with a bit of grated Parmesan cheese, if desired.

Nutritional Values

Please note that these are approximate values and may vary based on the exact measurements and specific ingredients used. This recipe serves 4.

Per serving:

Calories: 120
Total Fat: 10g
Saturated Fat: 6g
Total Carbohydrates: 5g (Net: 3g)
Protein: 4g

Health Benefits

High in Fiber: Both spinach and mushrooms are good sources of dietary fiber, which aids digestion and helps you feel full.
Rich in Antioxidants: Spinach is rich in antioxidants that can help protect your cells from damage.
Rich in Vitamins and Minerals: Spinach is a great source of vitamins A, C, K, and several B vitamins, as well as minerals such as calcium and iron. Mushrooms are a good source of B vitamins and minerals like selenium.
Anti-Inflammatory Properties: The antioxidants in spinach also have anti-inflammatory effects.
How it helps in Keto

This Spinach and Mushroom Sauté fits well into a keto diet as it is low in carbs and high in healthy fats from the butter or ghee. The spinach and mushrooms add fiber and bulk to the dish without adding many carbs, making it a satisfying meal that can help you stay within your daily carb limit.

Best time of the day to eat

This Keto Spinach and Mushroom Sauté can be enjoyed at any time of the day. It makes a delicious and nutritious breakfast, lunch, or dinner side dish. It could also be a main dish for lunch or dinner if paired with a protein source, such as a piece of grilled fish or chicken. As always, balance it with other meals to meet your daily macronutrient and calorie goals.

12 Keto Chia Pudding Recipe

Chia pudding is a versatile dish that can be eaten for breakfast, as a snack, or even dessert. Here's a simple, keto-friendly version that uses unsweetened almond milk and a touch of sweetener.

Ingredients

1/4 cup Chia Seeds
1 cup Unsweetened Almond Milk
1-2 tablespoons Erythritol or other low-carb sweetener
1/2 teaspoon Vanilla Extract
Toppings of choice: Berries, nuts, unsweetened coconut flakes, etc. (optional)

Instructions

- ➢ In a bowl, combine the chia seeds, unsweetened almond milk, erythritol, and vanilla extract. Stir well to combine.
- ➢ Let the mixture sit for about 5 minutes, then stir again to break up any clumps.
- ➢ Cover the bowl and refrigerate for at least 2 hours or overnight, until the mixture thickens to a pudding-like consistency.
- ➢ Before serving, stir the pudding well. If it's too thick, you can add a bit more almond milk.
- ➢ Serve the chia pudding with your favorite keto-friendly toppings, if desired.

Nutritional Values

Please note that these are approximate values and may vary based on the exact measurements and specific ingredients used. This recipe serves 2.

Per serving:

Calories: 145
Total Fat: 9g
Saturated Fat: 1g
Total Carbohydrates: 13g (Net: 2g, due to high fiber content)
Protein: 5g

Health Benefits

High in Fiber: Chia seeds are very high in fiber, which aids digestion and helps you feel full.
Rich in Omega-3 Fatty Acids: Chia seeds are a good source of Omega-3 fatty acids, which are beneficial for heart health.
Good Source of Minerals: Chia seeds provide important minerals like calcium, phosphorus, and manganese.
Antioxidants: Chia seeds are rich in antioxidants that can help protect your cells from damage.

How it helps in Keto

Keto Chia Pudding fits well into a keto diet as it is low in net carbs and high in fiber and healthy fats. The use of unsweetened almond milk and a low-carb sweetener keeps the carb content low.

Best time of the day to eat

This Keto Chia Pudding can be enjoyed at any time of the day, but it's particularly good as a start to your morning. It makes a quick and easy breakfast that you can prepare the night before. It can also serve as a snack or dessert. As always, balance it with other meals to meet your daily macronutrient and calorie goals.

13 Keto Tandoori Cauliflower Recipe

This keto-friendly recipe offers a flavorful and unique take on cauliflower by incorporating traditional Indian Tandoori spices.

Ingredients

1 medium Cauliflower, cut into florets
1 cup Greek Yogurt, unsweetened
2 tablespoons Tandoori Masala
1 teaspoon Turmeric Powder
1 teaspoon Cumin Powder
1 teaspoon Coriander Powder
Salt to taste
2 tablespoons Olive Oil
Fresh Cilantro for garnish

Instructions

➢ Preheat your oven to 400°F (200°C). Line a baking sheet with parchment paper.
➢ In a large bowl, combine the Greek yogurt, Tandoori Masala, turmeric powder, cumin powder, coriander powder, and salt. Mix until well combined.
➢ Add the cauliflower florets to the bowl and toss until they're coated with the yogurt mixture.
➢ Arrange the cauliflower florets in a single layer on the prepared baking sheet. Drizzle with the olive oil.
➢ Roast in the preheated oven for about 20-25 minutes, until the cauliflower is tender and the edges are browned.
➢ Garnish with fresh cilantro before serving.

Nutritional Values

Please note that these are approximate values and may vary based on the exact measurements and specific ingredients used. This recipe serves 4.

Calories: 140
Total Fat: 7g
Saturated Fat: 1g
Total Carbohydrates: 13g (Net: 9g)
Protein: 8g

Health Benefits

High in Fiber: Cauliflower is a good source of dietary fiber, which aids digestion and helps you feel full.
Rich in Antioxidants: Cauliflower, along with spices like turmeric, cumin, and coriander, are rich in antioxidants, which can help protect your cells from damage.
Anti-Inflammatory Properties: The curcumin in turmeric has powerful anti-inflammatory effects.
Rich in Vitamins and Minerals: Cauliflower is a good source of vitamins and minerals, such as vitamin C, vitamin K, and folate.

How it helps in Keto

Tandoori Cauliflower can fit well into a keto diet as it is relatively low in net carbs and high in fiber. The use of Greek yogurt and olive oil adds healthy fats to the meal. As with any keto meal, portion control is key to ensure you're staying within your daily carb limit.

Best time of the day to eat

This Keto Tandoori Cauliflower can be enjoyed as a main dish for lunch or dinner. It can be served with a side of cauliflower rice or a big green salad for a complete, keto-friendly meal. As always, balance it with other meals to meet your daily macronutrient and calorie goals.

14 Keto Masala Chai Recipe

Masala chai is a spiced tea beverage that originated from the Indian subcontinent. This keto-friendly version is made without milk and sugar, but still packs plenty of flavor.

Ingredients

2 cups of Water
2 Black Tea Bags
1 Cinnamon Stick
4 Green Cardamom Pods, crushed
2 Cloves
A small piece of fresh Ginger, crushed
1/2 cup of Heavy Cream or Coconut Milk (for a dairy-free option)
1-2 teaspoons of Erythritol or another keto-friendly sweetener

Instructions

- In a small saucepan, combine the water, tea bags, cinnamon stick, crushed cardamom pods, cloves, and crushed ginger.
- Bring the mixture to a boil over medium heat. Reduce the heat to low and let it simmer for about 10 minutes to let the spices infuse the tea.
- Remove the saucepan from heat and strain the tea into a cup or teapot to remove the spices and tea bags.
- Stir in the heavy cream or coconut milk, and the erythritol. You can return the tea to low heat for a minute or two if you want it hotter, but be careful not to let it boil.
- Serve the masala chai hot.

Nutritional Values

Please note that these are approximate values and may vary based on the exact measurements and specific ingredients used. This recipe serves 2.

Per serving:

Calories: 100
Total Fat: 10g
Saturated Fat: 7g
Total Carbohydrates: 3g (Net: 3g)
Protein: 1g

Health Benefits

Rich in Antioxidants: Black tea and spices like cinnamon, cardamom, cloves, and ginger are rich in antioxidants, which can help protect your cells from damage.
Anti-Inflammatory Properties: The spices used in masala chai have powerful anti-inflammatory effects.
Aids Digestion: Ginger and other spices can help to improve digestion.

How it helps in Keto

This Keto Masala Chai can fit well into a keto diet as it is low in carbs and provides some healthy fats from the heavy cream or coconut milk. Using a keto-friendly sweetener instead of sugar keeps the carb content low.

Best time of the day to eat

This Keto Masala Chai can be enjoyed at any time of the day, but it's particularly nice in the morning as a start to your day or in the afternoon as a pick-me-up. The warming spices make it a great beverage for a cold day. As always, balance it with other meals to meet your daily macronutrient and calorie goals.

15 Keto Cabbage Sabzi Recipe

Cabbage sabzi is a simple Indian stir-fry dish. This keto-friendly version is made with minimal spices to bring out the natural sweetness of the cabbage.

Ingredients

1 medium head of Cabbage, finely chopped
2 tablespoons of Coconut Oil or Ghee
1 teaspoon of Mustard Seeds
1 teaspoon of Cumin Seeds
1-2 Green Chilies, slit (optional, for heat)
A pinch of Asafoetida (Hing, optional)
Salt to taste
Fresh Cilantro for garnish

Instructions

- Heat the coconut oil or ghee in a large skillet or wok over medium heat.
- Add the mustard seeds and cumin seeds to the skillet. When they start to sputter, add the green chilies and asafoetida, if using.
- Add the chopped cabbage to the skillet. Stir well to combine with the spices and oil.
- Reduce the heat to medium-low, cover the skillet, and let the cabbage cook for about 10-15 minutes, stirring occasionally, until it's tender and lightly browned.
- Season with salt, stir well, and remove from heat.
- Garnish with fresh cilantro before serving.

Nutritional Values

Please note that these are approximate values and may vary based on the exact measurements and specific ingredients used. This recipe serves 4.

Per serving:

Calories: 110
Total Fat: 7g
Saturated Fat: 6g
Total Carbohydrates: 10g (Net: 6g)
Protein: 2g

Health Benefits

High in Fiber: Cabbage is a good source of dietary fiber, which aids digestion and helps you feel full.

Rich in Antioxidants: Cabbage is rich in antioxidants, including vitamin C and other phytonutrients, which can help protect your cells from damage.

Anti-Inflammatory Properties: Cabbage is known for its anti-inflammatory properties.

Rich in Vitamins and Minerals: Cabbage is a good source of vitamins K and C, and also provides some B vitamins and minerals like potassium and manganese.

How it helps in Keto

This Cabbage Sabzi fits well into a keto diet as it is low in net carbs and provides some healthy fats from the coconut oil or ghee. As with any keto meal, portion control is key to ensure you're staying within your daily carb limit.

Best time of the day to eat

This Keto Cabbage Sabzi can be enjoyed as a side dish for lunch or dinner. It pairs well with other Indian keto dishes, like paneer or a meat curry. As always, balance it with other meals to meet your daily macronutrient and calorie goals.

16 Keto Coconut Chutney Recipe

Coconut chutney is a popular South Indian condiment typically served with idli, dosa, and vada. Here's a keto-friendly version you can enjoy with keto breads or as a dip for vegetables.

Ingredients

1 cup of Fresh or Desiccated Coconut
2-3 Green Chilies
A small piece of Ginger
Salt to taste
1/2 cup of Water
For tempering: 1 tablespoon of Coconut Oil, 1/2 teaspoon of Mustard Seeds, a few Curry Leaves

Instructions

➢ In a blender or food processor, combine the coconut, green chilies, ginger, salt, and about half of the water. Blend until smooth, adding more water as needed to achieve your desired consistency.
➢ Transfer the chutney to a bowl.
➢ For the tempering, heat the coconut oil in a small skillet over medium heat. Add the mustard seeds and curry leaves. When the mustard seeds start to sputter, remove the skillet from heat.
➢ Pour the tempering over the chutney and stir to combine.
➢ Serve the chutney immediately, or refrigerate it for later use.

Nutritional Values

Please note that these are approximate values and may vary based on the exact measurements and specific ingredients used. This recipe serves 4.

Per serving:

Calories: 140
Total Fat: 13g
Saturated Fat: 11g
Total Carbohydrates: 6g (Net: 3g)
Protein: 1g

Health Benefits

Healthy Fats: Coconut is a great source of medium-chain triglycerides (MCTs), a type of fat that your body can use immediately for energy.
Rich in Fiber: Coconut also provides dietary fiber, which aids digestion and helps you feel full.
Antioxidants: Ingredients like green chilies and curry leaves provide antioxidants, which can help protect your cells from damage.

How it helps in Keto

This Coconut Chutney can fit well into a keto diet as it is low in net carbs and high in healthy fats from the coconut and coconut oil.

Best time of the day to eat

This Keto Coconut Chutney can be enjoyed at any time of the day as a condiment with your meals. It goes particularly well with keto breads or as a dip for vegetables. As always, balance it with other meals to meet your daily macronutrient and calorie goals.

17 Keto Matar Paneer Recipe

Matar Paneer is a classic Indian dish made with peas and paneer (Indian cheese) in a spicy tomato sauce. In this keto version, we will use low-carb vegetables instead of peas to maintain the original flavor while keeping it keto-friendly.

Ingredients

200 grams of Paneer, cubed
1 cup of Chopped Bell Peppers or Zucchini (as a low-carb replacement for peas)
1 Onion, finely chopped
2 Tomatoes, finely chopped
1 tablespoon of Ginger-Garlic Paste
2 tablespoons of Ghee or Coconut Oil
1 teaspoon of Cumin Seeds
1 teaspoon of Turmeric Powder
1 teaspoon of Red Chili Powder
1 teaspoon of Garam Masala
Salt to taste
Fresh Cilantro for garnish

Instructions

➢ Heat 1 tablespoon of ghee or coconut oil in a pan over medium heat. Add the paneer cubes and fry them until golden brown on all sides. Remove the paneer and set aside.

➢ In the same pan, add the remaining ghee or oil, then add the cumin seeds. Once they start to sputter, add the chopped onions and ginger-garlic paste. Sauté until the onions become translucent.

- ➢ Add the chopped tomatoes to the pan along with turmeric, red chili powder, and garam masala. Cook until the tomatoes are soft and the spices are well blended.
- ➢ Add the chopped bell peppers or zucchini to the pan and stir well. Cook for a few minutes until they are tender.
- ➢ Return the paneer to the pan, add salt, and mix well so that the paneer and vegetables are coated with the tomato-spice mixture.
- ➢ Cover the pan and let it simmer for 5-10 minutes.
- ➢ Garnish with fresh cilantro before serving.

Nutritional Values

Please note that these are approximate values and may vary based on the exact measurements and specific ingredients used. This recipe serves 4.

Per serving:

Calories: 250
Total Fat: 20g
Saturated Fat: 12g
Total Carbohydrates: 8g (Net: 5g)
Protein: 10g

Health Benefits

High in Protein: Paneer is a good source of protein, which is essential for muscle growth and repair.
Rich in Calcium: Paneer is also rich in calcium, which is important for bone health.
Rich in Vitamins and Minerals: Bell peppers or zucchini provide a range of vitamins and minerals, including vitamin C, potassium, and folate.

Anti-Inflammatory Properties: The spices used in matar paneer have powerful anti-inflammatory effects.

How it helps in Keto

This Keto Matar Paneer fits well into a keto diet as it is low in net carbs and high in fats from paneer and ghee. It also provides a moderate amount of protein, making it a balanced keto meal.

Best time of the day to eat

This Keto Matar Paneer can be enjoyed as a main dish for lunch or dinner. It pairs well with other Indian keto dishes, like cauliflower rice. As always, balance it with other meals to meet your daily macronutrient and calorie goals.

18 Keto Green Smoothie Recipe

This refreshing green smoothie is packed with nutritious, low-carb vegetables and healthy fats, making it an ideal choice for a keto diet.

Ingredients

1 cup of Spinach
1/2 an Avocado
1/2 a Cucumber
1/2 a cup of Unsweetened Almond Milk
A few Ice Cubes
Stevia or Erythritol to taste (optional)

Instructions

- ➤ Add all the ingredients into a blender.
- ➤ Blend until smooth. You can add more almond milk or water if it's too thick.
- ➤ Pour into a glass and enjoy immediately for the best taste and texture.

Nutritional Values

Please note that these are approximate values and may vary based on the exact measurements and specific ingredients used. This recipe serves 1.

Per serving:

Calories: 180
Total Fat: 15g

Saturated Fat: 2g
Total Carbohydrates: 12g (Net: 5g)
Protein: 4g

Health Benefits

High in Nutrients: This smoothie is packed with vitamins and minerals from the spinach, cucumber, and avocado. Spinach is rich in iron and vitamin K, cucumber provides hydration and vitamin C, and avocado is a great source of potassium and vitamin E.

Rich in Fiber: The vegetables and avocado in this smoothie provide dietary fiber, which aids digestion and helps you feel full.

Healthy Fats: Avocado and almond milk provide healthy monounsaturated fats, which are heart-healthy and can help to keep you satisfied.

How it helps in Keto

This Keto Green Smoothie can fit well into a keto diet as it is low in net carbs and high in healthy fats from the avocado and almond milk. The fiber in the vegetables and avocado also helps to reduce the net carb count.

Best time of the day to eat

This Keto Green Smoothie can be enjoyed at any time of the day, but it can be especially beneficial in the morning as a nutritious and quick breakfast option. It's also a great post-workout snack, providing hydration and a good mix of nutrients for recovery. As always, balance it with other meals to meet your daily macronutrient and calorie goals.

19 Keto Tomato Soup Recipe

A delicious and warming bowl of tomato soup can be easily made keto-friendly by using the right balance of ingredients.

Ingredients

4 cups of Fresh Tomatoes, chopped
1 Onion, chopped
2 cloves of Garlic, minced
1 tablespoon of Olive Oil or Coconut Oil
2 cups of Vegetable Broth
1 teaspoon of Dried Basil
Salt and Pepper to taste
1/2 cup of Heavy Cream
Fresh Basil for garnish

Instructions

➢ In a large pot, heat the oil over medium heat. Add the chopped onion and minced garlic and sauté until the onion is translucent.
➢ Add the chopped tomatoes to the pot along with the dried basil. Stir to combine with the onions and garlic and cook for a few minutes until the tomatoes start to break down.
➢ Add the vegetable broth to the pot and season with salt and pepper. Bring the mixture to a boil, then reduce the heat and let it simmer for about 20-30 minutes, until the tomatoes are very soft.
➢ Use an immersion blender to puree the soup until it's smooth. Alternatively, you can carefully transfer the soup to a countertop blender to puree it, then return it to the pot.

- ➢ Stir in the heavy cream and heat the soup for another few minutes until it's hot. Adjust the seasoning as needed.
- ➢ Serve the soup with a garnish of fresh basil.

Nutritional Values

Please note that these are approximate values and may vary based on the exact measurements and specific ingredients used. This recipe serves 4.

Per serving:

Calories: 200
Total Fat: 15g
Saturated Fat: 8g
Total Carbohydrates: 12g (Net: 8g)
Protein: 3g

Health Benefits

Rich in Vitamins: Tomatoes are a great source of vitamins C and K, as well as the antioxidant lycopene.
Heart Health: The olive oil or coconut oil and heavy cream provide heart-healthy monounsaturated fats.
Bone Health: The heavy cream provides a good amount of calcium, which is important for bone health.

How it helps in Keto

This Keto Tomato Soup fits well into a keto diet as it is low in net carbs and high in healthy fats from the oil and heavy cream.

Best time of the day to eat

This Keto Tomato Soup can be enjoyed as a light meal or snack at any time of the day. It's particularly nice for a warming lunch or dinner, especially on colder days. As always, balance it with other meals to meet your daily macronutrient and calorie goals.

20 Keto Paneer Tikka Recipe

Paneer Tikka is a popular Indian appetizer made from chunks of paneer (Indian cottage cheese) marinated in spices and grilled to perfection. In this keto-friendly version, we use high-fat paneer and a low-carb marinade.

Ingredients

200 grams of Paneer, cubed
2 tablespoons of Greek Yogurt
1 tablespoon of Olive Oil
1 teaspoon of Turmeric Powder
1 teaspoon of Red Chili Powder
1 teaspoon of Garam Masala
1 teaspoon of Cumin Powder
Salt to taste
1 tablespoon of Lemon Juice
Fresh Cilantro for garnish

Instructions

➢ In a bowl, combine the Greek yogurt, olive oil, turmeric powder, red chili powder, garam masala, cumin powder, salt, and lemon juice to make the marinade.

➢ Add the paneer cubes to the marinade and gently stir until all the paneer pieces are well-coated. Let it marinate for at least 30 minutes, but it's best if left for a few hours or overnight in the refrigerator.

➢ Preheat your grill or oven to a high temperature (about 200°C or 400°F).

- ➤ Skewer the marinated paneer pieces and grill them for about 15 minutes, or until they start to get a nice char. You can also bake them in the oven for about 20 minutes.
- ➤ Garnish with fresh cilantro and serve hot.

Nutritional Values

Please note that these are approximate values and may vary based on the exact measurements and specific ingredients used. This recipe serves 4.

Per serving:

Calories: 180
Total Fat: 15g
Saturated Fat: 7g
Total Carbohydrates: 3g (Net: 3g)
Protein: 8g

Health Benefits

High in Protein: Paneer is a good source of protein, which is essential for muscle growth and repair.
High in Calcium: Paneer is also rich in calcium, which is important for bone health.
Anti-Inflammatory Properties: The spices used in the marinade have anti-inflammatory effects and are packed with antioxidants.

How it helps in Keto

This Keto Paneer Tikka fits well into a keto diet as it is low in net carbs and high in fats from paneer and olive oil. It also provides a moderate amount of protein.

Best time of the day to eat

This Keto Paneer Tikka can be enjoyed as an appetizer or main dish for lunch or dinner. It pairs well with a salad or low-carb Indian breads like almond flour roti. As always, balance it with other meals to meet your daily macronutrient and calorie goals.

21 Keto Tofu Bhurji Recipe

Tofu Bhurji is a vegan version of the classic Indian scrambled dish. This keto-friendly version uses tofu, a low-carb, high-protein food that's a great plant-based option for a keto diet.

Ingredients

200 grams of Firm Tofu, crumbled
1 Onion, finely chopped
1 Tomato, finely chopped
2 Green Chilies, finely chopped
1 teaspoon of Turmeric Powder
1 teaspoon of Cumin Seeds
2 tablespoons of Olive Oil
Salt to taste
Fresh Cilantro for garnish

Instructions

➢ Heat the olive oil in a pan and add the cumin seeds. Once they start to splutter, add the chopped onion and green chilies.
➢ Sauté the onions and chilies until the onions become translucent. Then add the chopped tomatoes and cook until they become soft.
➢ Add the turmeric powder and salt to the pan and stir well.
➢ Crumble the tofu into the pan and mix well with the rest of the ingredients. Cook for about 5-10 minutes, until the tofu is well-cooked and has absorbed the flavors of the spices.
➢ Garnish with fresh cilantro and serve hot.

Nutritional Values

Please note that these are approximate values and may vary based on the exact measurements and specific ingredients used. This recipe serves 4.

Per serving:

Calories: 140
Total Fat: 10g
Saturated Fat: 1.5g
Total Carbohydrates: 5g (Net: 3g)
Protein: 8g
Health Benefits

High in Protein: Tofu is a great source of plant-based protein, which is essential for muscle growth and repair.
Good for Heart Health: Tofu contains isoflavones, which can help lower LDL cholesterol levels and reduce the risk of heart disease.
Rich in Nutrients: Tofu is a good source of iron, calcium, and other essential minerals.

How it helps in Keto

This Keto Tofu Bhurji is low in net carbs and high in protein, making it a good fit for a keto diet. The olive oil used for cooking also provides a good amount of healthy fats.

Best time of the day to eat

This Keto Tofu Bhurji can be enjoyed for breakfast, lunch, or dinner. It pairs well with a low-carb roti or as a filling in a lettuce wrap. As always, balance it with other meals to meet your daily macronutrient and calorie goals.

22 Keto Spiced Pumpkin Soup Recipe

Pumpkin soup is a classic fall dish, and this keto version is rich and creamy with a gentle hint of spice.

Ingredients

1 small Pumpkin, peeled and diced (about 4 cups)
2 tablespoons of Olive Oil
1 Onion, chopped
2 cloves of Garlic, minced
1 teaspoon of Ground Cinnamon
1/2 teaspoon of Ground Nutmeg
4 cups of Vegetable Broth
Salt and Pepper to taste
1/2 cup of Heavy Cream
Fresh Cilantro or Pumpkin Seeds for garnish

Instructions

➢ Heat the olive oil in a large pot over medium heat. Add the onion and garlic and sauté until the onion is translucent.

➢ Add the diced pumpkin, cinnamon, and nutmeg to the pot and stir to combine. Cook for a few minutes until the pumpkin begins to soften.

➢ Add the vegetable broth to the pot and season with salt and pepper. Bring the mixture to a boil, then reduce the heat and let it simmer for about 20 minutes, until the pumpkin is very soft.

➢ Use an immersion blender to puree the soup until it's smooth. Alternatively, you can carefully transfer the soup to a countertop blender to puree it, then return it to the pot.

- ➢ Stir in the heavy cream and heat the soup for another few minutes until it's hot. Adjust the seasoning as needed.
- ➢ Serve the soup with a garnish of fresh cilantro or pumpkin seeds.

Nutritional Values

Please note that these are approximate values and may vary based on the exact measurements and specific ingredients used. This recipe serves 4.

Per serving:

Calories: 280
Total Fat: 22g
Saturated Fat: 10g
Total Carbohydrates: 20g (Net: 14g)
Protein: 3g

Health Benefits

Rich in Vitamins: Pumpkin is a great source of vitamins A and C, both of which support a healthy immune system.
Heart Health: The olive oil and heavy cream provide heart-healthy monounsaturated fats.

How it helps in Keto

This Keto Spiced Pumpkin Soup fits well into a keto diet as it is low in net carbs and high in healthy fats from the oil and heavy cream.

Best time of the day to eat

This Keto Spiced Pumpkin Soup can be enjoyed as a light meal or snack at any time of the day. It's particularly nice for a warming lunch or dinner, especially on colder days. As always, balance it with other meals to meet your daily macronutrient and calorie goals.

23 Keto Baked Zucchini Recipe

Baked zucchini is a delicious and easy-to-make side dish that fits perfectly into a keto diet.

Ingredients

2 Zucchinis
2 tablespoons of Olive Oil
Salt and Pepper to taste
1/2 cup of Parmesan Cheese, grated
1/2 teaspoon of Garlic Powder
1/2 teaspoon of Italian Seasoning

Instructions

- ➢ Preheat your oven to 200°C (400°F) and line a baking sheet with parchment paper.
- ➢ Cut the zucchinis into half-inch thick rounds and arrange them on the baking sheet.
- ➢ Drizzle the zucchini rounds with olive oil and season with salt and pepper.
- ➢ In a small bowl, combine the grated parmesan, garlic powder, and Italian seasoning. Sprinkle this mixture evenly over the zucchini rounds.
- ➢ Bake for about 15-20 minutes, or until the zucchini is tender and the cheese is golden and bubbly.
- ➢ Serve hot.

Nutritional Values

Please note that these are approximate values and may vary based on the exact measurements and specific ingredients used. This recipe serves 4.

Per serving:

Calories: 130
Total Fat: 10g
Saturated Fat: 3g
Total Carbohydrates: 4g (Net: 3g)
Protein: 6g

Health Benefits

Low in Calories: Zucchini is a low-calorie vegetable that's also high in fiber, making it a great choice for weight loss.
High in Antioxidants: Zucchini is rich in antioxidants that can help protect your body from damage by free radicals.

How it helps in Keto

This Keto Baked Zucchini is low in net carbs and provides a good amount of healthy fats from the olive oil and cheese, which is ideal for a keto diet.

Best time of the day to eat

This Keto Baked Zucchini can be enjoyed as a side dish for lunch or dinner. It's also a great snack for those afternoon hunger pangs. As always, balance it with other meals to meet your daily macronutrient and calorie goals.

24 Keto Avocado Salad Recipe

Avocado salad is a fresh and vibrant dish that's loaded with healthy fats, making it perfect for a keto diet.

Ingredients

2 Avocados, peeled, pitted, and diced

1 Cucumber, diced

2 Tomatoes, diced

1/2 Onion, finely chopped

2 tablespoons of Olive Oil

1 tablespoon of Lemon Juice

Salt and Pepper to taste

Fresh Cilantro for garnish

Instructions

- ➤ In a large bowl, combine the diced avocados, cucumber, tomatoes, and chopped onion.
- ➤ In a small bowl, whisk together the olive oil and lemon juice. Season with salt and pepper.
- ➤ Pour the dressing over the salad and gently toss until everything is well-coated.
- ➤ Garnish with fresh cilantro and serve immediately.

Nutritional Values

Please note that these are approximate values and may vary based on the exact measurements and specific ingredients used. This recipe serves 4.

Per serving:

Calories: 250

Total Fat: 21g

Saturated Fat: 3g

Total Carbohydrates: 15g (Net: 6g)

Protein: 3g

Health Benefits

Heart Health: Avocados are rich in monounsaturated fats, which are heart-healthy. They also contain potassium, which can help control blood pressure.

Digestive Health: Avocados are a good source of dietary fiber, which supports a healthy digestive system.

How it helps in Keto

This Keto Avocado Salad is low in net carbs and high in healthy fats, which aligns with the nutritional needs of a ketogenic diet.

Best time of the day to eat

This Keto Avocado Salad is a versatile dish that can be enjoyed at any time of day. It's great for a light lunch or as a side dish for dinner. As always, balance it with other meals to meet your daily macronutrient and calorie goals.

25 Keto Lemon Rice Recipe

Lemon rice is a popular South Indian dish. This keto version uses cauliflower rice for a low-carb alternative.

Ingredients

4 cups of Cauliflower Rice

2 tablespoons of Olive Oil

1 teaspoon of Mustard Seeds

1/2 teaspoon of Turmeric Powder

1 Green Chili, finely chopped

Salt to taste

Juice of 1 Lemon

Fresh Cilantro for garnish

Instructions

- ➢ Heat the olive oil in a large pan over medium heat. Add the mustard seeds and let them splutter.
- ➢ Add the turmeric powder and chopped green chili to the pan and sauté for a few seconds.
- ➢ Add the cauliflower rice and salt to the pan and stir well. Cover the pan and let it cook for about 5-7 minutes, until the cauliflower rice is tender.
- ➢ Turn off the heat and add the lemon juice to the pan. Stir well to combine.

➢ Garnish with fresh cilantro and serve hot.

Nutritional Values

Please note that these are approximate values and may vary based on the exact measurements and specific ingredients used. This recipe serves 4.

Per serving:

Calories: 120

Total Fat: 7g

Saturated Fat: 1g

Total Carbohydrates: 12g (Net: 7g)

Protein: 4g

Health Benefits

Rich in Vitamins: Cauliflower is a great source of vitamins C and K, as well as other nutrients like folate.

Anti-inflammatory: Turmeric contains curcumin, which has potent anti-inflammatory properties.

How it helps in Keto

This Keto Lemon Rice is low in net carbs and has a moderate amount of healthy fats, which is suitable for a keto diet.

Best time of the day to eat

This Keto Lemon Rice can be enjoyed as a main dish for lunch or dinner. It's also great as a side dish with other low-carb Indian dishes. As always, balance it with other meals to meet your daily macronutrient and calorie goals.

26 Keto Cauliflower Pakora Recipe

Cauliflower pakora is a popular Indian snack. This keto version uses almond flour and flaxseed meal to keep it low-carb.

Ingredients

1 medium Cauliflower, cut into florets
1 cup of Almond Flour
2 tablespoons of Flaxseed Meal
1 teaspoon of Turmeric Powder
1 teaspoon of Chili Powder
Salt to taste
Water as needed
Olive Oil for frying

Instructions

➢ In a large bowl, combine the almond flour, flaxseed meal, turmeric powder, chili powder, and salt. Gradually add water, mixing until you get a thick batter.
➢ Dip each cauliflower floret into the batter, making sure it's well-coated.
➢ Heat the olive oil in a deep pan over medium heat. Once the oil is hot, carefully add the battered cauliflower florets, a few at a time.
➢ Fry the pakoras for a few minutes on each side, until they're golden brown and crispy.
➢ Remove the pakoras from the oil and drain on a paper towel-lined plate.
➢ Serve hot with a keto-friendly dipping sauce.

Nutritional Values

Please note that these are approximate values and may vary based on the exact measurements and specific ingredients used. This recipe serves 4.

Per serving:

Calories: 240
Total Fat: 20g
Saturated Fat: 2g
Total Carbohydrates: 10g (Net: 5g)
Protein: 8g

Health Benefits

Rich in Fiber: Almond flour and flaxseed meal are both high in fiber, which is beneficial for digestive health.
Heart Health: Olive oil and flaxseed are rich in monounsaturated fats and omega-3 fatty acids, which are good for heart health.

How it helps in Keto

These Keto Cauliflower Pakoras are low in net carbs and high in healthy fats, which makes them a great snack or appetizer for a keto diet.

Best time of the day to eat

These Keto Cauliflower Pakoras can be enjoyed as a snack at any time of day. They're particularly good for satisfying afternoon or evening cravings. As always, balance it with other meals to meet your daily macronutrient and calorie goals.

27 Keto Broccoli and Cheese Soup Recipe

Broccoli and cheese soup is a comforting and flavorful dish, and this keto version is both delicious and low in carbs.

Ingredients

2 cups of Broccoli Florets
1 small Onion, finely chopped
2 cloves of Garlic, minced
2 tablespoons of Butter or Olive Oil
3 cups of Vegetable or Chicken Broth
1 cup of Heavy Cream
1 cup of Shredded Cheddar Cheese
Salt and Pepper to taste

Instructions

➤ In a large pot, melt the butter or heat the olive oil over medium heat. Add the chopped onion and minced garlic and sauté until the onion is translucent.
➤ Add the broccoli florets to the pot and sauté for a few minutes until they start to soften.
➤ Pour in the vegetable or chicken broth and bring it to a boil. Reduce the heat and let it simmer for about 15 minutes, or until the broccoli is tender.
➤ Use an immersion blender or transfer the soup to a countertop blender to puree it until smooth.
➤ Return the soup to the pot and stir in the heavy cream. Heat the soup over low heat, then gradually add the shredded cheddar cheese while stirring continuously until it's fully melted and well incorporated.
➤ Season with salt and pepper to taste.

➤ Serve hot.

Nutritional Values

Please note that these are approximate values and may vary based on the exact measurements and specific ingredients used. This recipe serves 4.

Per serving:

Calories: 330
Total Fat: 28g
Saturated Fat: 17g
Total Carbohydrates: 7g (Net: 5g)
Protein: 10g

Health Benefits

High in Fiber: Broccoli is a great source of fiber, which aids digestion and promotes feelings of fullness.
Rich in Vitamins: Broccoli is packed with vitamins C, K, and folate, which are important for overall health and immune function.
Calcium and Protein: Cheddar cheese provides calcium and protein, which are essential for bone health and muscle repair.

How it helps in Keto

This Keto Broccoli and Cheese Soup is low in net carbs and high in healthy fats from the butter or olive oil, heavy cream, and cheese. It provides a moderate amount of protein.

Best time of the day to eat

This Keto Broccoli and Cheese Soup can be enjoyed as a meal on its own for lunch or dinner. It's especially comforting during colder months. As always, balance it with other meals to meet your daily macronutrient and calorie goals.

28 Keto Mushroom Soup Recipe

Mushroom soup is a rich and flavorful dish, and this keto version uses low-carb ingredients without sacrificing taste.

Ingredients

2 cups of Mushrooms, sliced
1 small Onion, finely chopped
2 cloves of Garlic, minced
2 tablespoons of Butter or Olive Oil
3 cups of Vegetable or Chicken Broth
1 cup of Heavy Cream
1 teaspoon of Thyme
Salt and Pepper to taste
Fresh Parsley for garnish

Instructions

➢ In a large pot, melt the butter or heat the olive oil over medium heat. Add the chopped onion and minced garlic and sauté until the onion is translucent.

➢ Add the sliced mushrooms to the pot and sauté until they release their moisture and start to brown.

➢ Pour in the vegetable or chicken broth and bring it to a boil. Reduce the heat and let it simmer for about 15 minutes, or until the mushrooms are tender.

➢ Use an immersion blender or transfer the soup to a countertop blender to puree it until smooth.

➢ Return the soup to the pot and stir in the heavy cream and thyme. Heat the soup over low heat for a few minutes until it's hot.

➢ Season with salt and pepper to taste.

➤ Garnish with fresh parsley and serve hot.

Nutritional Values

Please note that these are approximate values and may vary based on the exact measurements and specific ingredients used. This recipe serves 4.

Per serving:

Calories: 280
Total Fat: 25g
Saturated Fat: 15g
Total Carbohydrates: 8g (Net: 6g)
Protein: 4g

Health Benefits

Antioxidant-rich: Mushrooms are a great source of antioxidants, which help protect the body against free radicals.
Vitamin D: Mushrooms are one of the few natural sources of vitamin D, which is important for bone health and immune function.
Heart Health: The olive oil or butter and heavy cream provide heart-healthy monounsaturated fats.

How it helps in Keto

This Keto Mushroom Soup is low in net carbs and high in healthy fats from the butter or olive oil and heavy cream. It provides a moderate amount of protein.

Best time of the day to eat

This Keto Mushroom Soup can be enjoyed as a meal on its own for lunch or dinner. It's especially comforting during colder months.

29 Keto Spicy Grilled Eggplant Recipe

Spicy grilled eggplant is a flavorful and healthy dish that can be enjoyed as a side or as a light meal.

Ingredients

1 large Eggplant, sliced into rounds
2 tablespoons of Olive Oil
1 teaspoon of Paprika
1/2 teaspoon of Chili Powder
1/2 teaspoon of Cumin Powder
Salt and Pepper to taste
Fresh Cilantro or Mint for garnish

Instructions

➢ Preheat your grill or stovetop grill pan over medium-high heat.
➢ In a small bowl, combine the olive oil, paprika, chili powder, cumin powder, salt, and pepper to make the marinade.
➢ Brush both sides of the eggplant slices with the marinade.
➢ Grill the eggplant slices for about 3-4 minutes on each side, or until they are tender and have grill marks.
➢ Remove from the grill and garnish with fresh cilantro or mint.
➢ Serve hot.

Nutritional Values

Please note that these are approximate values and may vary based on the exact measurements and specific ingredients used. This recipe serves 4.

Per serving:

Calories: 80
Total Fat: 7g
Saturated Fat: 1g
Total Carbohydrates: 4g (Net: 2g)
Protein: 1g

Health Benefits

Low in Calories: Eggplant is low in calories, making it a great option for weight management.
Antioxidant-rich: Eggplant is rich in antioxidants, which help protect the body against damage from harmful free radicals.
Heart Health: Olive oil used in the marinade provides heart-healthy monounsaturated fats.

How it helps in Keto

This Keto Spicy Grilled Eggplant is low in net carbs and provides a moderate amount of healthy fats from the olive oil. It's a good option for a keto diet.

Best time of the day to eat

This Keto Spicy Grilled Eggplant can be enjoyed as a side dish for lunch or dinner. It pairs well with grilled meat or as part of a vegetarian meal. As always, balance it with other meals to meet your daily macronutrient and calorie goals.

30 Keto Masala Almonds Recipe

Masala almonds are a flavorful and crunchy snack that can be enjoyed on a keto diet.

Ingredients

1 cup of Almonds
1 tablespoon of Ghee or Olive Oil
1 teaspoon of Chili Powder
1/2 teaspoon of Turmeric Powder
1/2 teaspoon of Cumin Powder
1/4 teaspoon of Garam Masala
Salt to taste

Instructions

➢ Preheat your oven to 180°C (350°F) and line a baking sheet with parchment paper.
➢ In a bowl, combine the almonds, ghee or olive oil, chili powder, turmeric powder, cumin powder, garam masala, and salt. Toss well until the almonds are well-coated with the spices.
➢ Spread the seasoned almonds in a single layer on the prepared baking sheet.
➢ Bake for about 12-15 minutes, or until the almonds are toasted and fragrant. Stir the almonds halfway through baking to ensure even cooking.
➢ Remove from the oven and let the almonds cool completely before serving.

Nutritional Values

Please note that these are approximate values and may vary based on the exact measurements and specific ingredients used. This recipe serves 4.

Per serving:
Calories: 190
Total Fat: 17g
Saturated Fat: 2g
Total Carbohydrates: 6g (Net: 3g)
Protein: 6g

Health Benefits

Heart Health: Almonds are rich in monounsaturated fats, which are beneficial for heart health.
Vitamin E: Almonds are a good source of vitamin E, which acts as an antioxidant and supports healthy skin.
Minerals: Almonds are also rich in minerals such as magnesium, calcium, and potassium.

How it helps in Keto

These Keto Masala Almonds are low in net carbs and high in healthy fats, making them a great snack option for a keto diet.

Best time of the day to eat

These Keto Masala Almonds can be enjoyed as a snack at any time of the day. They're perfect for satisfying cravings or providing an energy boost between meals. As always, balance it with other meals to meet your daily macronutrient and calorie goals.

31 Keto Avocado Boats Recipe

Avocado boats are a delicious and nutritious way to enjoy the creamy goodness of avocados while following a keto diet.

Ingredients

2 Ripe Avocados
4-6 Cherry Tomatoes, halved
2 tablespoons of Feta Cheese, crumbled
2 tablespoons of Fresh Herbs (such as basil or cilantro), chopped
Salt and Pepper to taste
Optional toppings: Sliced Radishes, Sprouts, or Chopped Nuts

Instructions

➢ Cut the avocados in half lengthwise and remove the pits.
➢ Scoop out a little bit of flesh from the center of each avocado half to create a hollow for the filling.
➢ In a bowl, combine the cherry tomatoes, feta cheese, fresh herbs, salt, and pepper. Mix well.
➢ Spoon the tomato and cheese mixture into the hollowed-out center of each avocado half.
➢ Top with optional toppings if desired.
➢ Serve chilled.

Nutritional Values

Please note that these are approximate values and may vary based on the exact measurements and specific ingredients used. This recipe serves 2.

Per serving (1 avocado boat):

Calories: 230
Total Fat: 20g
Saturated Fat: 4g
Total Carbohydrates: 10g (Net: 2g)
Protein: 6g

Health Benefits

Healthy Fats: Avocados are rich in monounsaturated fats, which are good for heart health and help promote satiety.
Fiber: Avocados are also a good source of fiber, which aids digestion and promotes feelings of fullness.
Vitamins and Minerals: Avocados are packed with essential nutrients, including vitamins K, C, E, and B vitamins, as well as potassium and magnesium.

How it helps in Keto

These Keto Avocado Boats are low in net carbs and high in healthy fats, making them a great option for a keto diet. They provide a moderate amount of protein.

Best time of the day to eat

These Keto Avocado Boats can be enjoyed as a light meal or snack at any time of the day. They're perfect for a quick and satisfying lunch or as an appetizer before dinner. As always, balance it with other meals to meet your daily macronutrient and calorie goals.

32 Keto Cabbage Slaw Recipe

Cabbage slaw is a refreshing and crunchy side dish that can be enjoyed on a keto diet. It's packed with flavor and nutrients.

Ingredients

4 cups of Shredded Cabbage (green or purple)
1/2 cup of Shredded Carrots
1/4 cup of Chopped Red Onion
1/4 cup of Chopped Fresh Cilantro
2 tablespoons of Apple Cider Vinegar
2 tablespoons of Olive Oil
1 teaspoon of Dijon Mustard
Salt and Pepper to taste

Instructions

- ➢ In a large bowl, combine the shredded cabbage, shredded carrots, chopped red onion, and chopped cilantro.
- ➢ In a small bowl, whisk together the apple cider vinegar, olive oil, Dijon mustard, salt, and pepper to make the dressing.
- ➢ Pour the dressing over the cabbage mixture and toss well to combine.
- ➢ Let the slaw sit for at least 10 minutes before serving to allow the flavors to meld together.
- ➢ Serve chilled.

Nutritional Values

Please note that these are approximate values and may vary based on the exact measurements and specific ingredients used. This recipe serves 4.

Per serving:

Calories: 80
Total Fat: 6g
Saturated Fat: 1g
Total Carbohydrates: 6g (Net: 4g)
Protein: 1g

Health Benefits

Low in Calories: Cabbage is low in calories but high in fiber, making it a great choice for weight management.
Vitamins and Minerals: Cabbage is a good source of vitamin C, vitamin K, and other essential minerals.
Digestive Health: Cabbage contains fiber, which supports a healthy digestive system.

How it helps in Keto

This Keto Cabbage Slaw is low in net carbs and provides a moderate amount of healthy fats from the olive oil. It's a great option for a keto diet.

Best time of the day to eat

This Keto Cabbage Slaw can be enjoyed as a side dish for lunch or dinner. It pairs well with grilled meat or as part of a vegetarian meal. As always, balance it with other meals to meet your daily macronutrient and calorie goals.

33 Keto Palak Soup Recipe

Palak soup, also known as spinach soup, is a nutritious and flavorful dish that can be enjoyed as a light meal or as an appetizer.

Ingredients

4 cups of Fresh Spinach Leaves
1 small Onion, chopped
2 cloves of Garlic, minced
1/2 inch of Ginger, grated
2 cups of Vegetable Broth
1/2 cup of Heavy Cream
1 tablespoon of Ghee or Olive Oil
Salt and Pepper to taste
Fresh Lemon Juice for garnish (optional)

Instructions

➢ In a large pot, heat the ghee or olive oil over medium heat. Add the chopped onion, minced garlic, and grated ginger. Sauté until the onion becomes translucent.
➢ Add the spinach leaves to the pot and cook until wilted, about 2-3 minutes.
➢ Add the vegetable broth to the pot and bring it to a boil. Reduce the heat and let it simmer for about 10 minutes to allow the flavors to meld together.
➢ Use an immersion blender or transfer the soup to a countertop blender to puree it until smooth.
➢ Return the soup to the pot and stir in the heavy cream. Heat the soup over low heat for a few minutes until it's hot.
➢ Season with salt and pepper to taste.

> ➢ Serve hot, optionally with a squeeze of fresh lemon juice on top.

Nutritional Values

Please note that these are approximate values and may vary based on the exact measurements and specific ingredients used. This recipe serves 4.

Per serving:

Calories: 120
Total Fat: 11g
Saturated Fat: 7g
Total Carbohydrates: 4g (Net: 2g)
Protein: 3g

Health Benefits

Leafy Greens: Spinach is a nutrient-dense leafy green that provides vitamins A, C, and K, as well as iron and other minerals.
Antioxidants: Spinach is rich in antioxidants, which help protect the body against damage from harmful free radicals.
Heart Health: The ghee or olive oil and heavy cream provide heart-healthy fats.

How it helps in Keto

This Keto Palak Soup is low in net carbs and high in healthy fats from the ghee or olive oil and heavy cream. It's a good option for a keto diet.

Best time of the day to eat

This Keto Palak Soup can be enjoyed as a light meal or as an appetizer before a main course. It's particularly nice for a warming lunch or dinner, especially during colder months. As always, balance it with other meals to meet your daily macronutrient and calorie goals.

34 Keto Stuffed Mushrooms Recipe

Stuffed mushrooms make for a flavorful and satisfying appetizer or side dish, and this keto version is no exception.

Ingredients

12-15 Cremini or Button Mushrooms, stems removed
4 tablespoons of Cream Cheese, softened
2 tablespoons of Parmesan Cheese, grated
2 tablespoons of Almond Flour
1 clove of Garlic, minced
1 tablespoon of Fresh Parsley, chopped
Salt and Pepper to taste
Olive Oil for drizzling

Instructions

- ➤ Preheat your oven to 180°C (350°F) and line a baking sheet with parchment paper.
- ➤ In a bowl, combine the cream cheese, Parmesan cheese, almond flour, minced garlic, chopped parsley, salt, and pepper. Mix well until all the ingredients are fully incorporated.
- ➤ Place the mushroom caps on the prepared baking sheet, cavity side up.
- ➤ Spoon the cream cheese mixture into each mushroom cap, filling it generously.
- ➤ Drizzle a little bit of olive oil over each stuffed mushroom.
- ➤ Bake for about 15-20 minutes, or until the mushrooms are tender and the filling is golden brown.
- ➤ Remove from the oven and let the stuffed mushrooms cool for a few minutes before serving.

Nutritional Values

Please note that these are approximate values and may vary based on the exact measurements and specific ingredients used. This recipe serves 4.

Per serving (3-4 stuffed mushrooms):

Calories: 140
Total Fat: 12g
Saturated Fat: 5g
Total Carbohydrates: 4g (Net: 2g)
Protein: 6g

Health Benefits

Low in Carbs: Mushrooms are low in carbohydrates, making them a suitable choice for a keto diet.
Vitamins and Minerals: Mushrooms are a good source of B vitamins, selenium, and other minerals.
Healthy Fats: The cream cheese and olive oil provide a good amount of healthy fats.

How it helps in Keto

These Keto Stuffed Mushrooms are low in net carbs and provide a moderate amount of healthy fats from the cream cheese and olive oil. They're a great option for a keto-friendly appetizer or side dish.

Best time of the day to eat

These Keto Stuffed Mushrooms can be enjoyed as an appetizer before a meal or as a side dish. They're great for parties or gatherings. As always, balance it with other meals to meet your daily macronutrient and calorie goals.

35 Keto Lemon Rasam Recipe

Lemon rasam is a tangy and flavorful South Indian soup that can be enjoyed as an appetizer or as a light meal.

Ingredients

1 cup of Tamarind Extract
2 cups of Water
1 Tomato, chopped
1 small Onion, chopped
2 cloves of Garlic, minced
1/2 teaspoon of Turmeric Powder
1/2 teaspoon of Cumin Powder
1/2 teaspoon of Mustard Seeds
1/2 teaspoon of Fenugreek Seeds
1/4 teaspoon of Asafoetida (Hing)
2 tablespoons of Ghee or Coconut Oil
Juice of 1 Lemon
Salt to taste
Fresh Cilantro for garnish

Instructions

➢ In a large pot, combine the tamarind extract and water. Add the chopped tomato, chopped onion, minced garlic, turmeric powder, cumin powder, and salt. Bring the mixture to a boil.
➢ Reduce the heat and let it simmer for about 10 minutes, allowing the flavors to meld together.
➢ In a small pan, heat the ghee or coconut oil over medium heat. Add the mustard seeds, fenugreek seeds, and asafoetida. Let them splutter and become aromatic.

- ➤ Pour the tempered spices into the rasam pot and stir well.
- ➤ Add the lemon juice to the rasam and give it a final stir.
- ➤ Garnish with fresh cilantro before serving.

Nutritional Values

Please note that these are approximate values and may vary based on the exact measurements and specific ingredients used. This recipe serves 4.

Per serving:

Calories: 40
Total Fat: 4g
Saturated Fat: 2g
Total Carbohydrates: 3g (Net: 2g)
Protein: 1g

Health Benefits

Vitamin C: Lemon is a rich source of vitamin C, which is essential for a healthy immune system.
Digestive Health: Tamarind extract can aid digestion and promote a healthy gut.
Anti-inflammatory: Turmeric and cumin both have anti-inflammatory properties.

How it helps in Keto

This Keto Lemon Rasam is low in net carbs and provides a moderate amount of healthy fats from the ghee or coconut oil. It's a flavorful addition to a keto diet.

Best time of the day to eat

This Keto Lemon Rasam can be enjoyed as an appetizer before a meal or as a light meal itself. It's particularly soothing during colder months or when you need a tangy and refreshing flavor. As always, balance it with other meals to meet your daily macronutrient and calorie goals.

36 Keto Fried Okra Recipe

Fried okra is a crispy and delicious snack or side dish that can be enjoyed on a keto diet using low-carb breading.

Ingredients

2 cups of Okra, sliced into rounds
1/2 cup of Almond Flour
2 tablespoons of Coconut Flour
1/2 teaspoon of Paprika
1/2 teaspoon of Garlic Powder
Salt and Pepper to taste
2 Eggs, beaten
Olive Oil for frying

Instructions

➢ In a shallow bowl, combine the almond flour, coconut flour, paprika, garlic powder, salt, and pepper.
➢ Dip each okra slice into the beaten eggs, then coat it in the flour mixture, pressing lightly to ensure it's fully coated.
➢ Heat the olive oil in a large skillet over medium heat.
➢ Add the coated okra slices to the skillet in a single layer, making sure not to overcrowd the pan. Fry the okra for about 3-4 minutes on each side, or until they are golden brown and crispy.
➢ Remove the fried okra slices from the skillet and let them drain on a paper towel-lined plate.
➢ Serve hot.

Nutritional Values

Please note that these are approximate values and may vary based on the exact measurements and specific ingredients used. This recipe serves 4.

Per serving:

Calories: 170
Total Fat: 14g
Saturated Fat: 2g
Total Carbohydrates: 7g (Net: 4g)
Protein: 5g

Health Benefits

Fiber: Okra is a good source of fiber, which aids digestion and promotes feelings of fullness.
Vitamins and Minerals: Okra contains various vitamins and minerals, including vitamins A and C, folate, and potassium.

How it helps in Keto

This Keto Fried Okra is low in net carbs and provides a moderate amount of healthy fats from the olive oil and almond flour coating. It's a great option for a keto-friendly snack or side dish.

Best time of the day to eat

This Keto Fried Okra can be enjoyed as a snack or as a side dish for lunch or dinner. It's particularly delicious when served hot and crispy. As always, balance it with other meals to meet your daily macronutrient and calorie goals.

37 Keto Cheese Stuffed Jalapenos Recipe

Keto cheese-stuffed jalapenos are a delicious and spicy appetizer that can be enjoyed on a keto diet. The combination of jalapeno peppers and gooey cheese creates a flavor-packed bite.

Ingredients

8-10 Jalapeno Peppers
4 ounces of Cream Cheese, softened
1/2 cup of Shredded Cheddar Cheese
1/4 cup of Finely Chopped Bacon (optional)
Salt and Pepper to taste

Instructions

- ➢ Preheat your oven to 180°C (350°F) and line a baking sheet with parchment paper.
- ➢ Cut the jalapeno peppers in half lengthwise and remove the seeds and membranes, keeping the stem intact for a nice presentation.
- ➢ In a bowl, combine the cream cheese, shredded cheddar cheese, chopped bacon (if using), salt, and pepper. Mix well until all the ingredients are fully incorporated.
- ➢ Spoon the cheese mixture into each jalapeno half, filling it generously.
- ➢ Place the stuffed jalapeno halves on the prepared baking sheet.
- ➢ Bake for about 15-20 minutes, or until the jalapenos are tender and the cheese is melted and slightly golden.
- ➢ Remove from the oven and let the stuffed jalapenos cool for a few minutes before serving.

Nutritional Values

Please note that these are approximate values and may vary based on the exact measurements and specific ingredients used. This recipe serves 4.

Per serving (2-3 stuffed jalapeno halves):

Calories: 120
Total Fat: 10g
Saturated Fat: 6g
Total Carbohydrates: 2g (Net: 1g)
Protein: 5g

Health Benefits

Capsaicin: Jalapenos contain capsaicin, a compound that gives them their spicy flavor and has been shown to have anti-inflammatory and metabolism-boosting properties.
Vitamin C: Jalapenos are a good source of vitamin C, which supports a healthy immune system.
Calcium and Protein: Cheese is rich in calcium and protein, which are important for bone health and muscle function.

How it helps in Keto

These Keto Cheese Stuffed Jalapenos are low in net carbs and high in healthy fats from the cheese and cream cheese. They provide a moderate amount of protein.

Best time of the day to eat

These Keto Cheese Stuffed Jalapenos can be enjoyed as an appetizer before a meal or as a snack. They're perfect for parties or gatherings. As always, balance it with other meals to meet your daily macronutrient and calorie goals.

38 Keto Bhindi Masala Recipe

Bhindi masala is a flavorful Indian dish made with okra and a blend of spices. This keto version omits any high-carb ingredients to make it suitable for a keto diet.

Ingredients

2 cups of Okra, chopped into bite-sized pieces
1 Onion, finely chopped
2 Tomatoes, finely chopped
2 tablespoons of Ghee or Coconut Oil
1 teaspoon of Cumin Seeds
1/2 teaspoon of Turmeric Powder
1/2 teaspoon of Red Chili Powder
1/2 teaspoon of Coriander Powder
1/4 teaspoon of Garam Masala
Salt to taste
Fresh Cilantro for garnish

Instructions

➢ Heat the ghee or coconut oil in a pan over medium heat. Add the cumin seeds and let them splutter.
➢ Add the chopped onions to the pan and sauté until they turn golden brown.
➢ Add the chopped tomatoes to the pan and cook until they soften and release their juices.
➢ Add the turmeric powder, red chili powder, coriander powder, and salt. Mix well to coat the onions and tomatoes with the spices.

- ➤ Add the chopped okra to the pan and mix it with the onion and tomato mixture. Cook for about 10-12 minutes, stirring occasionally, until the okra is tender.
- ➤ Sprinkle garam masala over the cooked bhindi masala and give it a final stir.
- ➤ Garnish with fresh cilantro before serving.

Nutritional Values

Please note that these are approximate values and may vary based on the exact measurements and specific ingredients used. This recipe serves 4.

Per serving:

Calories: 90
Total Fat: 7g
Saturated Fat: 5g
Total Carbohydrates: 6g (Net: 3g)
Protein: 2g

Health Benefits

Fiber: Okra is a good source of fiber, which aids digestion and promotes feelings of fullness.

Vitamins and Minerals: Okra contains various vitamins and minerals, including vitamins A and C, folate, and potassium.

Antioxidants: The spices used in the bhindi masala, such as turmeric and chili powder, contain antioxidants that have potential health benefits.

How it helps in Keto

This Keto Bhindi Masala is low in net carbs and provides a moderate amount of healthy fats from the ghee or coconut oil. It's a flavorful option for a keto-friendly Indian dish.

Best time of the day to eat

This Keto Bhindi Masala can be enjoyed as a side dish for lunch or dinner. It pairs well with other Indian dishes or can be served with keto-friendly bread or cauliflower rice. As always, balance it with other meals to meet your daily macronutrient and calorie goals.

39 Keto Tomato Bharta Recipe

Tomato bharta is a delicious Indian dish made with roasted tomatoes and a blend of spices. This keto version eliminates any high-carb ingredients to make it suitable for a keto diet.

Ingredients

4 Tomatoes
1 Onion, finely chopped
2 cloves of Garlic, minced
1 Green Chili Pepper, finely chopped (optional)
1/2 teaspoon of Cumin Seeds
1/2 teaspoon of Turmeric Powder
1/2 teaspoon of Red Chili Powder
1/2 teaspoon of Garam Masala
2 tablespoons of Ghee or Coconut Oil
Salt to taste
Fresh Cilantro for garnish

Instructions

- Preheat your oven to 200°C (400°F). Place the tomatoes on a baking sheet and roast them for about 20-25 minutes or until the skin starts to blister and peel.
- Remove the tomatoes from the oven and let them cool. Peel off the skin and roughly chop the roasted tomatoes.
- Heat the ghee or coconut oil in a pan over medium heat. Add the cumin seeds and let them splutter.
- Add the chopped onions to the pan and sauté until they turn golden brown.
- Add the minced garlic and chopped green chili pepper (if using) to the pan. Sauté for another minute.

- ➢ Add the turmeric powder, red chili powder, and salt. Mix well to coat the onions and spices.
- ➢ Add the roasted and chopped tomatoes to the pan. Mix everything together and cook for about 5-7 minutes, allowing the flavors to meld together.
- ➢ Sprinkle garam masala over the cooked tomato bharta and give it a final stir.
- ➢ Garnish with fresh cilantro before serving.

Nutritional Values

Please note that these are approximate values and may vary based on the exact measurements and specific ingredients used. This recipe serves 4.

Per serving:

Calories: 50
Total Fat: 4g
Saturated Fat: 3g
Total Carbohydrates: 4g (Net: 2g)
Protein: 1g

Health Benefits

Lycopene: Tomatoes are rich in lycopene, an antioxidant that may help reduce the risk of certain diseases.
Vitamins and Minerals: Tomatoes are a good source of vitamins A and C, as well as potassium.
Antioxidants: The spices used in the tomato bharta, such as turmeric and chili powder, contain antioxidants that have potential health benefits.

How it helps in Keto

This Keto Tomato Bharta is low in net carbs and provides a moderate amount of healthy fats from the ghee or coconut oil. It's a flavorful option for a keto-friendly Indian dish.

Best time of the day to eat

This Keto Tomato Bharta can be enjoyed as a side dish for lunch or dinner. It pairs well with other Indian dishes or can be served with keto-friendly bread or cauliflower rice. As always, balance it with other meals to meet your daily macronutrient and calorie goals.

40 Keto Creamy Tomato Basil Soup Recipe

Creamy tomato basil soup is a comforting and flavorful dish that can be enjoyed on a keto diet. This version eliminates any high-carb ingredients to make it keto-friendly.

Ingredients

4 Tomatoes, chopped
1/2 Onion, chopped
2 cloves of Garlic, minced
1 cup of Vegetable Broth
1/2 cup of Heavy Cream
2 tablespoons of Tomato Paste
2 tablespoons of Fresh Basil, chopped
1 tablespoon of Olive Oil
Salt and Pepper to taste

Instructions

➢ In a large pot, heat the olive oil over medium heat. Add the chopped onion and minced garlic. Sauté until the onion becomes translucent.

➢ Add the chopped tomatoes to the pot and cook until they soften and release their juices.

➢ Add the vegetable broth, tomato paste, salt, and pepper. Bring the mixture to a boil, then reduce the heat and let it simmer for about 15-20 minutes, allowing the flavors to meld together.

➢ Use an immersion blender or transfer the soup to a countertop blender to puree it until smooth.

- ➤ Return the soup to the pot and stir in the heavy cream and chopped basil. Heat the soup over low heat for a few minutes until it's hot.
- ➤ Season with additional salt and pepper if needed.
- ➤ Serve hot.

Nutritional Values

Please note that these are approximate values and may vary based on the exact measurements and specific ingredients used. This recipe serves 4.

Per serving:

Calories: 170
Total Fat: 13g
Saturated Fat: 7g
Total Carbohydrates: 8g (Net: 5g)
Protein: 3g

Health Benefits

Vitamins and Minerals: Tomatoes are a good source of vitamins A and C, as well as potassium.
Antioxidants: Tomatoes and basil contain antioxidants that have potential health benefits.
Healthy Fats: The heavy cream and olive oil provide a good amount of healthy fats.

How it helps in Keto

This Keto Creamy Tomato Basil Soup is low in net carbs and high in healthy fats from the heavy cream and olive oil. It's a comforting and satisfying option for a keto-friendly soup.

Best time of the day to eat

This Keto Creamy Tomato Basil Soup can be enjoyed as a light meal or as an appetizer before a main course. It's particularly comforting during colder months or when you're craving a warm and creamy soup. As always, balance it with other meals to meet your daily macronutrient and calorie goals.

41 Keto Roasted Cauliflower Recipe

Roasted cauliflower is a versatile and delicious side dish that can be enjoyed on a keto diet. It's simple to prepare and brings out the natural sweetness of the cauliflower.

Ingredients

1 head of Cauliflower, cut into florets
2 tablespoons of Olive Oil
1 teaspoon of Garlic Powder
1/2 teaspoon of Paprika
Salt and Pepper to taste
Fresh Parsley for garnish (optional)

Instructions

➢ Preheat your oven to 200°C (400°F) and line a baking sheet with parchment paper.
➢ In a large bowl, toss the cauliflower florets with olive oil, garlic powder, paprika, salt, and pepper. Make sure the florets are well coated with the seasoning.
➢ Spread the cauliflower florets in a single layer on the prepared baking sheet.
➢ Roast in the preheated oven for about 20-25 minutes, or until the cauliflower is tender and golden brown, tossing once halfway through.
➢ Remove from the oven and let the roasted cauliflower cool for a few minutes.
➢ Garnish with fresh parsley before serving.

Nutritional Values

Please note that these are approximate values and may vary based on the exact measurements and specific ingredients used. This recipe serves 4.

Per serving:

Calories: 80
Total Fat: 6g
Saturated Fat: 1g
Total Carbohydrates: 6g (Net: 4g)
Protein: 2g

Health Benefits

Fiber: Cauliflower is a good source of fiber, which aids digestion and promotes feelings of fullness.
Vitamins and Minerals: Cauliflower contains various vitamins and minerals, including vitamins C and K, folate, and potassium.
Antioxidants: Cauliflower is rich in antioxidants, which help protect the body against damage from harmful free radicals.

How it helps in Keto

This Keto Roasted Cauliflower is low in net carbs and provides a moderate amount of healthy fats from the olive oil. It's a versatile and nutritious option for a keto-friendly side dish.

Best time of the day to eat

This Keto Roasted Cauliflower can be enjoyed as a side dish for lunch or dinner. It pairs well with a variety of main courses and can be used in salads or bowls. As always, balance it with other meals to meet your daily macronutrient and calorie goals.

42 Keto Roasted Brussels Sprouts Recipe

Roasted Brussels sprouts are a flavorful and nutritious side dish that can be enjoyed on a keto diet. Roasting brings out their natural sweetness and adds a delicious caramelized flavor.

Ingredients

2 cups of Brussels Sprouts, trimmed and halved
2 tablespoons of Olive Oil
2 cloves of Garlic, minced
Salt and Pepper to taste
Lemon Juice (optional)

Instructions

➢ Preheat your oven to 200°C (400°F) and line a baking sheet with parchment paper.
➢ In a bowl, toss the Brussels sprouts with olive oil, minced garlic, salt, and pepper. Make sure the sprouts are well coated with the seasoning.
➢ Spread the Brussels sprouts in a single layer on the prepared baking sheet.
➢ Roast in the preheated oven for about 20-25 minutes, or until the sprouts are tender and lightly browned, tossing once halfway through.
➢ Remove from the oven and drizzle with a little bit of lemon juice, if desired, for a fresh citrus flavor.
➢ Let the roasted Brussels sprouts cool for a few minutes before serving.

Nutritional Values

Please note that these are approximate values and may vary based on the exact measurements and specific ingredients used. This recipe serves 4.

Per serving:

Calories: 90
Total Fat: 7g
Saturated Fat: 1g
Total Carbohydrates: 7g (Net: 4g)
Protein: 3g

Health Benefits

Fiber: Brussels sprouts are a good source of fiber, which aids digestion and promotes feelings of fullness.
Vitamins and Minerals: Brussels sprouts are rich in vitamins C and K, as well as folate and potassium.
Antioxidants: Brussels sprouts contain antioxidants, which help protect the body against damage from harmful free radicals.

How it helps in Keto

This Keto Roasted Brussels Sprouts recipe is low in net carbs and provides a moderate amount of healthy fats from the olive oil. It's a nutritious and flavorful option for a keto-friendly side dish.

Best time of the day to eat

This Keto Roasted Brussels Sprouts can be enjoyed as a side dish for lunch or dinner. They pair well with a variety of main courses and can be incorporated into salads or bowls. As always, balance it with other meals to meet your daily macronutrient and calorie goals.

43 Keto Paneer Makhani Recipe

Paneer makhani is a rich and creamy Indian dish made with paneer (Indian cottage cheese) and a flavorful tomato-based sauce. This keto version omits any high-carb ingredients to make it suitable for a keto diet.

Ingredients

200g Paneer, cut into cubes
4 Tomatoes, pureed
1/2 cup of Heavy Cream
2 tablespoons of Ghee or Coconut Oil
1 teaspoon of Ginger-Garlic Paste
1/2 teaspoon of Turmeric Powder
1/2 teaspoon of Red Chili Powder
1/2 teaspoon of Garam Masala
Salt to taste
Fresh Cilantro for garnish

Instructions

➢ In a pan, heat the ghee or coconut oil over medium heat. Add the ginger-garlic paste and sauté until fragrant.
➢ Add the pureed tomatoes to the pan and cook until the raw smell of the tomatoes goes away and the mixture thickens.
➢ Add the turmeric powder, red chili powder, garam masala, and salt. Mix well to combine the spices with the tomato mixture.
➢ Reduce the heat to low and add the heavy cream. Stir well to incorporate the cream into the sauce.

- ➢ Add the paneer cubes to the pan and gently mix them with the sauce. Cook for a few minutes, allowing the flavors to meld together and the paneer to absorb the sauce.
- ➢ Garnish with fresh cilantro before serving.

Nutritional Values

Please note that these are approximate values and may vary based on the exact measurements and specific ingredients used. This recipe serves 4.

Per serving:

Calories: 280
Total Fat: 24g
Saturated Fat: 15g
Total Carbohydrates: 7g (Net: 5g)
Protein: 10g

Health Benefits

Protein: Paneer is a good source of protein, which is essential for muscle growth and repair.
Calcium: Paneer is rich in calcium, which is important for maintaining strong bones and teeth.
Vitamins and Minerals: Tomatoes used in the sauce are a good source of vitamins A and C, as well as potassium.

How it helps in Keto

This Keto Paneer Makhani is low in net carbs and provides a moderate amount of healthy fats from the ghee or coconut oil and heavy cream. It's a flavorful and satisfying option for a keto-friendly Indian dish.

Best time of the day to eat

This Keto Paneer Makhani can be enjoyed as a main course for lunch or dinner. It pairs well with keto-friendly bread or cauliflower rice. As always, balance it with other meals to meet your daily macronutrient and calorie goals.

44 Keto Spicy Roasted Almonds Recipe

Spicy roasted almonds are a crunchy and flavorful snack that can be enjoyed on a keto diet. They're easy to make and perfect for satisfying those snack cravings.

Ingredients

1 cup of Raw Almonds
1 tablespoon of Olive Oil
1 teaspoon of Paprika
1/2 teaspoon of Cayenne Pepper
1/2 teaspoon of Garlic Powder
1/2 teaspoon of Salt
1/4 teaspoon of Black Pepper

Instructions

➤ Preheat your oven to 180°C (350°F) and line a baking sheet with parchment paper.
➤ In a bowl, combine the raw almonds, olive oil, paprika, cayenne pepper, garlic powder, salt, and black pepper. Toss well to ensure the almonds are evenly coated with the seasoning.
➤ Spread the seasoned almonds in a single layer on the prepared baking sheet.
➤ Roast in the preheated oven for about 10-15 minutes, or until the almonds are toasted and fragrant.
➤ Remove from the oven and let the roasted almonds cool completely before storing them in an airtight container.

Nutritional Values

Please note that these are approximate values and may vary based on the exact measurements and specific ingredients used. This recipe yields approximately 4 servings.

Per serving (1/4 cup):

Calories: 180
Total Fat: 16g
Saturated Fat: 1g
Total Carbohydrates: 5g (Net: 3g)
Protein: 7g

Health Benefits

Healthy Fats: Almonds are a good source of healthy fats, including monounsaturated fats and omega-3 fatty acids, which are beneficial for heart health.
Protein: Almonds provide a moderate amount of protein, which is important for various functions in the body.
Vitamins and Minerals: Almonds contain various vitamins and minerals, including vitamin E, magnesium, and calcium.

How it helps in Keto

These Keto Spicy Roasted Almonds are low in net carbs and provide a good amount of healthy fats and protein. They make for a satisfying and crunchy keto-friendly snack.

Best time of the day to eat

These Keto Spicy Roasted Almonds can be enjoyed as a snack between meals or incorporated into your meal plan as an ingredient in salads or other dishes. As always, balance it with other meals to meet your daily macronutrient and calorie goals.

45 Keto Green Bean Salad Recipe

Green bean salad is a refreshing and nutritious dish that can be enjoyed on a keto diet. It's packed with fresh flavors and provides a good amount of fiber and vitamins.

Ingredients

2 cups of Green Beans, trimmed and halved
1/4 cup of Red Onion, thinly sliced
1/4 cup of Cherry Tomatoes, halved
2 tablespoons of Olive Oil
1 tablespoon of Lemon Juice
1 tablespoon of Fresh Parsley, chopped
Salt and Pepper to taste

Instructions

- Fill a pot with water and bring it to a boil. Add the green beans to the boiling water and cook for about 2-3 minutes, or until they are tender-crisp.
- Drain the green beans and immediately transfer them to a bowl of ice water to stop the cooking process and preserve their vibrant green color. Let them cool for a few minutes, then drain.
- In a large bowl, combine the blanched green beans, red onion, cherry tomatoes, olive oil, lemon juice, chopped parsley, salt, and pepper. Toss well to coat the ingredients with the dressing.
- Let the salad marinate in the refrigerator for at least 30 minutes before serving, allowing the flavors to meld together.
- Serve chilled.

Nutritional Values

Please note that these are approximate values and may vary based on the exact measurements and specific ingredients used. This recipe serves 4.

Per serving:

Calories: 90
Total Fat: 7g
Saturated Fat: 1g
Total Carbohydrates: 5g (Net: 3g)
Protein: 2g

Health Benefits

Fiber: Green beans are a good source of fiber, which aids digestion and promotes feelings of fullness.
Vitamins and Minerals: Green beans contain various vitamins and minerals, including vitamins A, C, and K, as well as folate and potassium.
Antioxidants: Green beans are rich in antioxidants, which help protect the body against damage from harmful free radicals.

How it helps in Keto

This Keto Green Bean Salad is low in net carbs and provides a moderate amount of healthy fats from the olive oil. It's a refreshing and nutrient-dense option for a keto-friendly salad.

Best time of the day to eat

This Keto Green Bean Salad can be enjoyed as a side dish for lunch or dinner. It pairs well with grilled chicken, fish, or other protein sources. As always, balance it with other meals to meet your daily macronutrient and calorie goals.

46 Keto Zucchini Spaghetti Recipe

Zucchini spaghetti, also known as zoodles, is a low-carb and gluten-free alternative to traditional pasta. It's light, flavorful, and perfect for a keto diet.

Ingredients

2 medium-sized Zucchini
2 tablespoons of Olive Oil
2 cloves of Garlic, minced
Salt and Pepper to taste
Fresh Basil or Parsley for garnish (optional)

Instructions

> Using a spiralizer or vegetable peeler, cut the zucchini into long, thin strands resembling spaghetti noodles. If using a spiralizer, follow the manufacturer's instructions.
> Heat the olive oil in a large pan over medium heat. Add the minced garlic and sauté until fragrant.
> Add the zucchini noodles to the pan and toss gently to coat them with the garlic-infused oil. Cook for about 2-3 minutes, or until the zucchini noodles are tender but still have a slight crunch.
> Season the zucchini spaghetti with salt and pepper to taste.
> Remove from heat and garnish with fresh basil or parsley, if desired.

Nutritional Values

Please note that these are approximate values and may vary based on the exact measurements and specific ingredients used. This recipe serves 2.

Per serving:

Calories: 100
Total Fat: 7g
Saturated Fat: 1g
Total Carbohydrates: 6g (Net: 4g)
Protein: 3g

Health Benefits

Low Carb: Zucchini is low in carbs, making it a suitable substitute for traditional pasta on a keto diet.
Fiber: Zucchini contains fiber, which aids digestion and promotes feelings of fullness.
Vitamins and Minerals: Zucchini is a good source of vitamins A and C, as well as potassium.

How it helps in Keto

This Keto Zucchini Spaghetti is very low in net carbs and provides a moderate amount of healthy fats from the olive oil. It's a light and satisfying option for a keto-friendly pasta substitute.

Best time of the day to eat

This Keto Zucchini Spaghetti can be enjoyed as a main course for lunch or dinner. It can be served with a variety of keto-friendly sauces, such as tomato-based or pesto sauces, and topped with protein sources such as grilled chicken or shrimp. As always, balance it with other meals to meet your daily macronutrient and calorie goals.

47 Keto Cauliflower Fried Rice

Cauliflower fried rice is a delicious and low-carb alternative to traditional fried rice. It replaces rice with cauliflower, making it suitable for a keto diet. Here's how you can make it:

Ingredients:

1 head of Cauliflower, riced (you can use a food processor or grate it with a box grater)
2 tablespoons of Sesame Oil
2 cloves of Garlic, minced
1 small Onion, diced
1 cup of Mixed Vegetables (such as carrots, peas, and bell peppers)
2 Eggs, beaten
2 tablespoons of Soy Sauce (or Tamari for gluten-free)
Salt and Pepper to taste
Optional toppings: Green onions, Sesame seeds

Instructions:

- ➤ Heat the sesame oil in a large skillet or wok over medium heat.
- ➤ Add the minced garlic and diced onion to the pan and sauté until they become fragrant and the onion turns translucent.
- ➤ Add the mixed vegetables to the pan and cook until they are slightly tender.
- ➤ Push the vegetables to one side of the pan and pour the beaten eggs onto the other side. Scramble the eggs until they are cooked through.
- ➤ Mix the scrambled eggs with the vegetables and add the riced cauliflower to the pan. Stir-fry everything together for

a few minutes, until the cauliflower is cooked but still has a slight crunch.

Drizzle the soy sauce over the cauliflower fried rice and season with salt and pepper to taste. Stir well to combine all the ingredients and evenly distribute the flavors.

Remove from heat and garnish with green onions and sesame seeds, if desired.

Nutritional Values:

Please note that these values are approximate and may vary based on specific ingredients used and serving size.

Per serving (1/4 of the recipe):

Calories: 150
Total Fat: 8g
Saturated Fat: 1g
Total Carbohydrates: 14g (Net: 7g)
Fiber: 7g
Protein: 8g

Health Benefits:

Low-Carb: Cauliflower is a low-carb vegetable and serves as a great substitute for rice in this dish.

Fiber: Cauliflower is high in fiber, which promotes healthy digestion and helps maintain stable blood sugar levels.

Vitamins and Minerals: Cauliflower is rich in vitamins C, K, and B6, as well as folate and potassium.

How it Helps in Keto:

Cauliflower fried rice is a keto-friendly dish because it replaces high-carb rice with low-carb cauliflower. It provides a satisfying and flavorful alternative for those following a keto diet.

Best Time of the Day to Eat:

You can enjoy keto cauliflower fried rice as a main course for lunch or dinner. It can be paired with a protein source, such as grilled chicken or tofu, to make it a complete meal. As always, balance it with other meals to meet your daily macronutrient and calorie goals.

48 Keto Avocado Cucumber Salad

Avocado cucumber salad is a refreshing and nutritious dish that fits well into a keto diet. It's packed with healthy fats and fresh flavors. Here's how you can make it:

Ingredients:

1 large Avocado, diced
1 medium Cucumber, peeled and diced
1/4 Red Onion, thinly sliced
1 tablespoon of Fresh Cilantro, chopped
Juice of 1/2 Lemon
2 tablespoons of Olive Oil
Salt and Pepper to taste

Instructions:

- ➤ In a large bowl, combine the diced avocado, cucumber, red onion, and chopped cilantro.
- ➤ Drizzle the lemon juice and olive oil over the ingredients.
- ➤ Season with salt and pepper to taste.
- ➤ Gently toss everything together until well combined.
- ➤ Let the salad sit for a few minutes to allow the flavors to meld together.
- ➤ Serve chilled.

Nutritional Values:

Please note that these values are approximate and may vary based on specific ingredients used and serving size.

Per serving (1/2 of the recipe):

Calories: 220
Total Fat: 20g
Saturated Fat: 3g
Total Carbohydrates: 10g (Net: 5g)
Fiber: 5g
Protein: 2g

Health Benefits:

Healthy Fats: Avocado is a great source of healthy monounsaturated fats, which are beneficial for heart health.
Hydration: Cucumbers are high in water content, helping to keep you hydrated.
Vitamins and Minerals: Avocado and cucumber are rich in vitamins C, K, and E, as well as potassium and magnesium.

How it Helps in Keto:

Avocado cucumber salad is a keto-friendly dish that provides a good amount of healthy fats and fiber while being low in net carbs. It's a satisfying and nutritious option for those following a keto diet.

Best Time of the Day to Eat:

You can enjoy avocado cucumber salad as a side dish for lunch or dinner. It pairs well with grilled meat or fish. It can also be a refreshing and filling option for a light meal during hot summer days. As always, balance it with other meals to meet your daily macronutrient and calorie goals.

49 Keto Creamy Spinach Soup

Creamy spinach soup is a nutritious and comforting dish that can be enjoyed on a keto diet. It's rich in flavor and packed with healthy ingredients. Here's how you can make it:

Ingredients:

4 cups of Fresh Spinach, washed and roughly chopped
1 small Onion, diced
2 cloves of Garlic, minced
2 tablespoons of Butter or Olive Oil
2 cups of Vegetable or Chicken Broth
1 cup of Heavy Cream
Salt and Pepper to taste
Optional toppings: Grated Parmesan cheese, Crumbled bacon

Instructions:

➤ In a large pot, melt the butter or heat the olive oil over medium heat.
➤ Add the diced onion and minced garlic to the pot and sauté until they become fragrant and the onion turns translucent.
➤ Add the chopped spinach to the pot and cook until it wilts down, stirring occasionally.
➤ Pour in the vegetable or chicken broth and bring it to a simmer. Let it cook for about 10 minutes to allow the flavors to meld together.
➤ Using an immersion blender or a regular blender, blend the soup until smooth and creamy. Be careful when blending hot liquids.
➤ Return the soup to the pot and stir in the heavy cream. Season with salt and pepper to taste.

- ➢ Simmer the soup for an additional 5 minutes to heat it through.
- ➢ Remove from heat and serve hot.
- ➢ Garnish with grated Parmesan cheese or crumbled bacon, if desired.

Nutritional Values:

Please note that these values are approximate and may vary based on specific ingredients used and serving size.

Per serving (1/4 of the recipe):

Calories: 220
Total Fat: 19g
Saturated Fat: 12g
Total Carbohydrates: 7g (Net: 3g)
Fiber: 4g
Protein: 5g

Health Benefits:

Iron and Calcium: Spinach is a good source of iron and calcium, important minerals for overall health.

Vitamins and Antioxidants: Spinach is rich in vitamins A, C, and K, as well as antioxidants that help protect the body against damage from harmful free radicals.

Healthy Fats: The heavy cream provides healthy fats, which are beneficial for a ketogenic diet.

How it Helps in Keto:

Keto creamy spinach soup is low in net carbs and high in healthy fats, making it a suitable choice for those following a keto diet.

It provides a comforting and nutrient-rich option for a keto-friendly soup.

Best Time of the Day to Eat:

You can enjoy creamy spinach soup as a starter or main course for lunch or dinner. It pairs well with a side salad or a protein source, such as grilled chicken or fish. As always, balance it with other meals to meet your daily macronutrient and calorie goals.

50 Keto Garlic Roasted Broccoli

Garlic roasted broccoli is a flavorful and nutritious side dish that can be enjoyed on a keto diet. Roasting brings out the natural sweetness of the broccoli while adding a hint of garlic. Here's how you can make it:

Ingredients:

1 large head of Broccoli, cut into florets
2 tablespoons of Olive Oil
3 cloves of Garlic, minced
Salt and Pepper to taste
Optional toppings: Grated Parmesan cheese, Lemon zest

Instructions:

➢ Preheat your oven to 200°C (400°F) and line a baking sheet with parchment paper.
➢ In a large bowl, toss the broccoli florets with olive oil, minced garlic, salt, and pepper. Make sure the florets are well coated with the seasoning.
➢ Spread the broccoli florets in a single layer on the prepared baking sheet.
➢ Roast In the preheated oven for about 20-25 minutes, or until the florets are tender and lightly browned, tossing once halfway through.
➢ Remove from the oven and sprinkle with grated Parmesan cheese or lemon zest, if desired, for added flavor.
➢ Let the roasted broccoli cool for a few minutes before serving.

Nutritional Values:

Please note that these values are approximate and may vary based on specific ingredients used and serving size.

Per serving (1/4 of the recipe):

Calories: 90
Total Fat: 7g
Saturated Fat: 1g
Total Carbohydrates: 7g (Net: 4g)
Fiber: 3g
Protein: 3g

Health Benefits:

Vitamins and Minerals: Broccoli is a nutrient-dense vegetable, rich in vitamins C, K, and folate, as well as minerals such as potassium and calcium.
Fiber: Broccoli is high in fiber, promoting healthy digestion and aiding in weight management.
Antioxidants: Broccoli contains antioxidants, which help protect the body against damage from harmful free radicals.

How it Helps in Keto:

Garlic roasted broccoli is low in net carbs and provides a moderate amount of healthy fats from the olive oil. It's a flavorful and nutritious option for a keto-friendly side dish.

Best Time of the Day to Eat:

You can enjoy garlic roasted broccoli as a side dish for lunch or dinner. It pairs well with a variety of main courses and can be incorporated into salads or bowls. As always, balance it with other meals to meet your daily macronutrient and calorie goals.

51 Keto Tandoori Tofu

Tandoori tofu is a flavorful and protein-packed dish that can be enjoyed on a keto diet. It's marinated in a blend of aromatic spices and then grilled or baked to perfection. Here's how you can make it:

Ingredients:

1 block of Firm Tofu, drained and pressed
2 tablespoons of Greek Yogurt (or coconut yogurt for dairy-free)
1 tablespoon of Lemon Juice
2 teaspoons of Tandoori Masala Spice Blend
1 teaspoon of Paprika
1/2 teaspoon of Ground Cumin
1/2 teaspoon of Ground Coriander
1/2 teaspoon of Turmeric
1/2 teaspoon of Salt
1/4 teaspoon of Cayenne Pepper (adjust to taste)
2 tablespoons of Olive Oil (for grilling or baking)
Fresh Cilantro for garnish (optional)
Lemon wedges for serving

Instructions:

➢ Cut the tofu into cubes or slices, depending on your preference.
➢ In a bowl, combine the Greek yogurt, lemon juice, tandoori masala spice blend, paprika, ground cumin, ground coriander, turmeric, salt, and cayenne pepper. Mix well to create a smooth marinade.
➢ Add the tofu to the marinade and gently toss until each piece is evenly coated. Allow the tofu to marinate for at

least 30 minutes, or longer for more intense flavor. You can marinate it in the refrigerator overnight if desired.

- ➤ If grilling: Preheat your grill to medium-high heat. Thread the tofu onto skewers or use a grill basket to prevent it from falling through the grates. Grill for about 4-5 minutes on each side, or until the tofu is nicely charred and heated through.
- ➤ If baking: Preheat your oven to 200°C (400°F). Line a baking sheet with parchment paper. Place the marinated tofu in a single layer on the baking sheet and bake for 20-25 minutes, flipping halfway through, or until the tofu is crispy and golden.
- ➤ Remove the tofu from the grill or oven and let it cool slightly.
- ➤ Garnish with fresh cilantro, if desired, and serve with lemon wedges for squeezing over the tofu.

Nutritional Values:

Please note that these values are approximate and may vary based on specific ingredients used and serving size.

Per serving (1/4 of the recipe):

Calories: 150
Total Fat: 11g
Saturated Fat: 2g
Total Carbohydrates: 6g (Net: 4g)
Fiber: 2g
Protein: 10g

Health Benefits:

Protein: Tofu is a plant-based protein source, providing all essential amino acids necessary for muscle growth and repair.

Soy Isoflavones: Tofu contains isoflavones, which have been associated with various health benefits, including reducing the risk of heart disease.

Antioxidants: The spices used in tandoori tofu, such as turmeric and cayenne pepper, contain antioxidants that help protect the body against damage from harmful free radicals.

How it Helps in Keto:

Tandoori tofu is low in net carbs and provides a good amount of protein. It can be enjoyed as a main course or added to salads or wraps, offering a delicious and satisfying option for those following a keto diet.

Best Time of the Day to Eat:

You can enjoy tandoori tofu as a main course for lunch or dinner. Serve it with a side of grilled vegetables or a fresh salad for a complete meal. As always, balance it with other meals to meet your daily macronutrient and calorie goals.

52 Keto Aloo Gobi (using cauliflower instead of potatoes)

Aloo Gobi is a classic Indian dish that traditionally consists of potatoes and cauliflower. In this keto-friendly version, we replace the potatoes with cauliflower to make it low in carbs. Here's how you can make it:

Ingredients:

1 small head of Cauliflower, cut into florets
1 small Onion, finely chopped
2 cloves of Garlic, minced
1 teaspoon of Ginger, grated
1 small Tomato, finely chopped
1/2 teaspoon of Turmeric
1/2 teaspoon of Cumin Powder
1/2 teaspoon of Coriander Powder
1/4 teaspoon of Red Chili Powder (adjust to taste)
1/4 teaspoon of Garam Masala
2 tablespoons of Ghee or Coconut Oil
Fresh Cilantro for garnish (optional)
Salt to taste

Instructions:

➢ Heat the ghee or coconut oil in a large skillet or pan over medium heat.
➢ Add the chopped onion and sauté until it becomes translucent.
➢ Add the minced garlic and grated ginger to the pan. Sauté for another minute until fragrant.

- ➢ Add the chopped tomato and cook until it softens and breaks down.
- ➢ Stir in the turmeric, cumin powder, coriander powder, red chili powder, and salt. Mix well to coat the onions and tomatoes with the spices.
- ➢ Add the cauliflower florets to the pan and mix everything together, ensuring the florets are coated with the spice mixture.
- ➢ Reduce the heat to low, cover the pan, and let the cauliflower cook for about 10-15 minutes, or until it is tender. Stir occasionally to prevent sticking.
- ➢ Once the cauliflower is cooked, sprinkle garam masala over it and give it a final stir.
- ➢ Remove from heat and garnish with fresh cilantro, if desired.

Nutritional Values:

Please note that these values are approximate and may vary based on specific ingredients used and serving size.

Per serving (1/4 of the recipe):

Calories: 80
Total Fat: 7g
Saturated Fat: 4g
Total Carbohydrates: 5g (Net: 3g)
Fiber: 2g
Protein: 2g

Health Benefits:

Low-Carb: By using cauliflower instead of potatoes, this dish becomes low in carbohydrates, making it suitable for a keto diet.

Fiber: Cauliflower is a good source of fiber, which aids digestion and helps maintain stable blood sugar levels.

Vitamins and Minerals: Cauliflower is rich in vitamins C, K, and B6, as well as folate and potassium.

How it Helps in Keto:

Keto Aloo Gobi is a flavorful and satisfying dish that is low in net carbs and provides a moderate amount of healthy fats from the ghee or coconut oil. It's a great option for those following a keto diet.

Best Time of the Day to Eat:

You can enjoy Keto Aloo Gobi as a main course for lunch or dinner. Serve it with a side of raita (yogurt-based dip) or keto-friendly flatbread for a complete meal. As always, balance it with other meals to meet your daily macronutrient and calorie goals.

53 Keto Spiced Pumpkin Seeds

Spiced pumpkin seeds are a crunchy and flavorful snack that can be enjoyed on a keto diet. They are rich in healthy fats and provide a good amount of protein. Here's how you can make them:

Ingredients:

1 cup of Pumpkin Seeds (pepitas)

1 tablespoon of Olive Oil or Melted Butter

1/2 teaspoon of Salt

1/2 teaspoon of Smoked Paprika

1/4 teaspoon of Garlic Powder

1/4 teaspoon of Onion Powder

1/4 teaspoon of Cayenne Pepper (adjust to taste)

Instructions:

➢ Preheat your oven to 150°C (300°F) and line a baking sheet with parchment paper.

➢ In a bowl, combine the pumpkin seeds, olive oil or melted butter, salt, smoked paprika, garlic powder, onion powder, and cayenne pepper. Mix well to ensure the seeds are evenly coated with the spices.

➢ Spread the seasoned pumpkin seeds in a single layer on the prepared baking sheet.

➢ Roast in the preheated oven for about 25-30 minutes, stirring once or twice during baking, until the pumpkin seeds are golden brown and crispy.

➢ Remove from the oven and let the spiced pumpkin seeds cool completely before transferring them to an airtight container for storage.

Nutritional Values:

Please note that these values are approximate and may vary based on specific ingredients used and serving size.

Per serving (1/4 cup):

Calories: 180
Total Fat: 16g
Saturated Fat: 3g
Total Carbohydrates: 2g (Net: 1g)
Fiber: 1g
Protein: 9g

Health Benefits:

Healthy Fats: Pumpkin seeds are a good source of healthy fats, including omega-3 fatty acids, which are beneficial for heart health.
Protein: Pumpkin seeds are rich in protein, which is essential for muscle growth and repair.
Minerals: Pumpkin seeds are a good source of minerals, including magnesium, zinc, and iron.

How it Helps in Keto:

Spiced pumpkin seeds are a nutritious and satisfying snack option for those following a keto diet. They are low in net carbs and provide a good amount of healthy fats and protein.

Best Time of the Day to Eat:

You can enjoy spiced pumpkin seeds as a snack between meals or add them to salads or trail mixes for an extra crunch. They can also be used as a topping for soups or roasted vegetables.

As always, balance them with other meals to meet your daily macronutrient and calorie goals.

54 Keto Eggplant Parmesan

Eggplant Parmesan is a classic Italian dish that is typically breaded and fried. In this keto-friendly version, we skip the breading and use low-carb ingredients to create a delicious and healthier alternative. Here's how you can make it:

Ingredients:

1 large Eggplant, sliced into 1/2-inch thick rounds
Salt, for sweating the eggplant
Olive Oil, for brushing
1 cup of Low-carb Marinara Sauce
1 cup of Shredded Mozzarella Cheese
1/4 cup of Grated Parmesan Cheese
Fresh Basil leaves, for garnish (optional)

Instructions:

➤ Preheat your oven to 200°C (400°F) and line a baking sheet with parchment paper.
➤ Place the eggplant slices on a paper towel-lined surface and sprinkle them with salt. Let them sit for about 20-30 minutes to draw out excess moisture.
➤ After 30 minutes, pat the eggplant slices dry with paper towels to remove the salt and moisture.
➤ Brush both sides of the eggplant slices with olive oil and place them on the prepared baking sheet.
➤ Roast in the preheated oven for about 15-20 minutes, flipping halfway through, until the eggplant is tender and lightly golden.
➤ Remove the eggplant slices from the oven and spoon a layer of marinara sauce over each slice.

- ➢ Sprinkle shredded mozzarella cheese and grated Parmesan cheese over the sauce.
- ➢ Return the baking sheet to the oven and broil for about 3-5 minutes, or until the cheese is melted and bubbly.
- ➢ Remove from the oven and let it cool slightly before serving.
- ➢ Garnish with fresh basil leaves, if desired.

Nutritional Values:

Please note that these values are approximate and may vary based on specific ingredients used and serving size.

Per serving (1/4 of the recipe):

Calories: 180
Total Fat: 12g
Saturated Fat: 6g
Total Carbohydrates: 9g (Net: 6g)
Fiber: 3g
Protein: 9g

Health Benefits:

Low-Carb: By omitting the breading and using low-carb ingredients, this keto Eggplant Parmesan is lower in carbohydrates compared to the traditional version.
Antioxidants: Eggplant is rich in antioxidants, which help protect the body against damage from harmful free radicals.
Vitamins and Minerals: Eggplant is a good source of vitamins C, K, and B6, as well as minerals like potassium and magnesium.

How it Helps in Keto:

Keto Eggplant Parmesan is a flavorful and satisfying dish that is low in net carbs and provides a moderate amount of healthy fats from the olive oil and cheese. It's a great option for those following a keto diet.

Best Time of the Day to Eat:

You can enjoy Keto Eggplant Parmesan as a main course for lunch or dinner. Serve it with a side of fresh salad or roasted vegetables for a complete meal. As always, balance it with other meals to meet your daily macronutrient and calorie goals.

55 Keto Zucchini Chips

Zucchini chips are a tasty and low-carb alternative to traditional potato chips. They are crispy, flavorful, and easy to make. Here's how you can make them:

Ingredients:

2 medium Zucchini, sliced into thin rounds
2 tablespoons of Olive Oil
Salt and Pepper to taste
Optional seasonings: Garlic powder, Onion powder, Paprika, Italian seasoning, etc.

Instructions:

- ➤ Preheat your oven to 120°C (250°F) and line a baking sheet with parchment paper.
- ➤ Place the zucchini slices in a large bowl and drizzle with olive oil. Toss to coat the slices evenly.
- ➤ Arrange the zucchini slices in a single layer on the prepared baking sheet.
- ➤ Sprinkle salt, pepper, and any optional seasonings of your choice over the zucchini slices.
- ➤ Bake in the preheated oven for about 1 to 1 1/2 hours, or until the zucchini slices are crispy and golden brown, flipping them once halfway through.
- ➤ Keep an eye on them during the last few minutes to prevent burning.
- ➤ Remove from the oven and let the zucchini chips cool completely before serving.

Nutritional Values:

Please note that these values are approximate and may vary based on specific ingredients used and serving size.

Per serving (1/4 of the recipe):

Calories: 90
Total Fat: 7g
Saturated Fat: 1g
Total Carbohydrates: 4g (Net: 2g)
Fiber: 2g
Protein: 2g

Health Benefits:

Low-Carb and Low-Calorie: Zucchini is low in carbs and calories, making it a suitable choice for keto diets.
Vitamins and Minerals: Zucchini is a good source of vitamins A, C, and K, as well as minerals like potassium and magnesium.
Antioxidants: Zucchini contains antioxidants, which help protect the body against damage from harmful free radicals.

How it Helps in Keto:

Zucchini chips are a delicious and satisfying snack that is low in net carbs and provides a moderate amount of healthy fats from the olive oil. They are a great option for satisfying your craving for crunchy snacks while following a keto diet.

Best Time of the Day to Eat:

You can enjoy zucchini chips as a snack between meals or as a side dish for lunch or dinner. They pair well with dips such as guacamole or sour cream. As always, balance them with other meals to meet your daily macronutrient and calorie goals.

56 Keto Cabbage Stir Fry

Cabbage stir fry is a quick and flavorful dish that can be enjoyed on a keto diet. It's a versatile recipe that allows you to incorporate various low-carb vegetables and protein sources. Here's a basic recipe to get you started:

Ingredients:

4 cups of Shredded Cabbage (green or Napa cabbage)
1 small Onion, sliced
2 cloves of Garlic, minced
1 small Carrot, julienned
1/2 Red Bell Pepper, sliced
2 tablespoons of Soy Sauce (or tamari for gluten-free)
1 tablespoon of Sesame Oil
1 tablespoon of Olive Oil
Salt and Pepper to taste
Optional protein sources: Tofu, Chicken, Shrimp, etc.

Instructions:

➢ Heat the olive oil and sesame oil in a large skillet or wok over medium-high heat.
➢ Add the minced garlic to the pan and sauté for about 30 seconds until fragrant.
➢ Add the sliced onion, julienned carrot, and sliced bell pepper to the pan. Stir-fry for about 2-3 minutes until the vegetables start to soften.
➢ If using protein sources like tofu, chicken, or shrimp, add them to the pan and cook until they are cooked through.

➤ Add the shredded cabbage to the pan and continue stir-frying for another 3-4 minutes until the cabbage is slightly wilted but still crisp.
➤ Stir in the soy sauce (or tamari) and season with salt and pepper to taste. Toss everything together until well combined.
➤ Remove from heat and serve hot.

Nutritional Values:

Please note that these values are approximate and may vary based on specific ingredients used and serving size.

Per serving (1/4 of the recipe):

Calories: 90
Total Fat: 6g
Saturated Fat: 1g
Total Carbohydrates: 7g (Net: 5g)
Fiber: 2g
Protein: 2g

Health Benefits:

Low-Carb and Low-Calorie: Cabbage is low in carbs and calories, making it a suitable choice for keto diets.
Fiber: Cabbage is rich in fiber, which promotes healthy digestion and aids in weight management.
Vitamins and Minerals: Cabbage is a good source of vitamins C, K, and B6, as well as minerals like potassium and calcium.

How it Helps in Keto:

Cabbage stir fry is a nutritious and satisfying dish that is low in net carbs and provides a moderate amount of healthy fats from the oils used. It's a great way to incorporate low-carb vegetables into your keto diet.

Best Time of the Day to Eat:

You can enjoy cabbage stir fry as a side dish or main course for lunch or dinner. It pairs well with a variety of protein sources and can be customized with your favorite low-carb vegetables. As always, balance it with other meals to meet your daily macronutrient and calorie goals.

57 Keto Spinach and Cheese Stuffed Mushrooms

Spinach and cheese stuffed mushrooms are a delicious and satisfying appetizer or side dish that is perfect for a keto diet. Here's how you can make them:

Ingredients:

12 large Cremini or Button Mushrooms
1 cup of Fresh Spinach, chopped
1/2 cup of Shredded Mozzarella Cheese
1/4 cup of Grated Parmesan Cheese
2 tablespoons of Cream Cheese
1 clove of Garlic, minced
1 tablespoon of Olive Oil
Salt and Pepper to taste
Fresh Parsley for garnish (optional)

Instructions:

➢ Preheat your oven to 200°C (400°F) and line a baking sheet with parchment paper.
➢ Remove the stems from the mushrooms and set them aside. Place the mushroom caps on the prepared baking sheet, stem side up.
➢ Finely chop the reserved mushroom stems.
➢ In a skillet, heat the olive oil over medium heat. Add the chopped mushroom stems and minced garlic to the skillet. Sauté for 3-4 minutes until the moisture from the mushrooms evaporates.
➢ Add the chopped spinach to the skillet and cook for an additional 2 minutes until it wilts.

- ➢ Remove the skillet from heat and let the mixture cool slightly.
- ➢ In a bowl, combine the sautéed mushroom and spinach mixture with shredded mozzarella cheese, grated Parmesan cheese, cream cheese, salt, and pepper. Mix well to combine.
- ➢ Spoon the filling into each mushroom cap, pressing it down gently.
- ➢ Bake in the preheated oven for about 15-20 minutes, or until the mushrooms are tender and the cheese is melted and slightly golden.
- ➢ Remove from the oven and let the stuffed mushrooms cool for a few minutes before serving.
- ➢ Garnish with fresh parsley, if desired.

Nutritional Values:

Please note that these values are approximate and may vary based on specific ingredients used and serving size.

Per serving (3 stuffed mushrooms):

Calories: 120
Total Fat: 9g
Saturated Fat: 4g
Total Carbohydrates: 3g (Net: 2g)
Fiber: 1g
Protein: 7g

Health Benefits:

Spinach: Spinach is packed with vitamins A, C, and K, as well as minerals like iron and magnesium.

Cheese: The combination of mozzarella and Parmesan cheese provides calcium and protein, which are important for bone health and muscle maintenance.

Mushrooms: Mushrooms are low in calories and carbohydrates while being a good source of fiber and various nutrients, including vitamin D and selenium.

How it Helps in Keto:

Spinach and cheese stuffed mushrooms are low in net carbs and provide a good amount of healthy fats and protein. They can be enjoyed as an appetizer or side dish on a keto diet.

Best Time of the Day to Eat:

You can enjoy spinach and cheese stuffed mushrooms as a snack or appetizer before a meal. They can also be served as a side dish alongside a protein source for a complete keto-friendly meal. As always, balance them with other meals to meet your daily macronutrient and calorie goals.

58 Keto Roasted Eggplant

Roasted eggplant is a versatile and delicious dish that can be enjoyed as a side dish or incorporated into other keto recipes. Here's how you can make it:

Ingredients:

1 large Eggplant
2 tablespoons of Olive Oil
Salt and Pepper to taste
Optional seasonings: Garlic powder, Paprika, Italian seasoning, etc.

Instructions:

- ➢ Preheat your oven to 200°C (400°F) and line a baking sheet with parchment paper.
- ➢ Wash the eggplant and trim off the stem. Cut it into 1/2-inch thick rounds or lengthwise slices, depending on your preference.
- ➢ Place the eggplant slices on a paper towel-lined surface and sprinkle them with salt. Let them sit for about 20-30 minutes to draw out excess moisture.
- ➢ After 30 minutes, pat the eggplant slices dry with paper towels to remove the salt and moisture.
- ➢ Place the eggplant slices on the prepared baking sheet and brush both sides with olive oil.
- ➢ Sprinkle salt, pepper, and any optional seasonings of your choice over the eggplant slices.
- ➢ Roast in the preheated oven for about 20-25 minutes, flipping them halfway through, until the eggplant is tender and golden brown.

➤ Remove from the oven and let the roasted eggplant cool slightly before serving.

Nutritional Values:

Please note that these values are approximate and may vary based on specific ingredients used and serving size.

Per serving (1/4 of the recipe):

Calories: 80
Total Fat: 7g
Saturated Fat: 1g
Total Carbohydrates: 4g (Net: 2g)
Fiber: 2g
Protein: 1g

Health Benefits:

Eggplant: Eggplant is low in calories and carbohydrates while being a good source of dietary fiber. It also contains antioxidants that help protect against cellular damage.
Olive Oil: Olive oil provides healthy monounsaturated fats, which have been linked to various health benefits, including heart health and reduced inflammation.

How it Helps in Keto:

Roasted eggplant is low in net carbs and provides a moderate amount of healthy fats. It can be enjoyed as a side dish or used as a base for other keto recipes.

Best Time of the Day to Eat:

Roasted eggplant can be enjoyed as a side dish for lunch or dinner. It pairs well with grilled meats or can be used as a topping for salads or in keto-friendly wraps. As always, balance it with other meals to meet your daily macronutrient and calorie goals.

59 Keto Curry Roasted Cauliflower

Curry roasted cauliflower is a flavorful and satisfying dish that can be enjoyed as a side or main course on a keto diet. Here's how you can make it:

Ingredients:

1 large head of Cauliflower, cut into florets
2 tablespoons of Olive Oil
1 tablespoon of Curry Powder
1 teaspoon of Paprika
1/2 teaspoon of Turmeric
1/2 teaspoon of Cumin
1/2 teaspoon of Garlic Powder
Salt and Pepper to taste
Fresh Cilantro for garnish (optional)

Instructions:

➢ Preheat your oven to 200°C (400°F) and line a baking sheet with parchment paper.
➢ In a large bowl, combine the olive oil, curry powder, paprika, turmeric, cumin, garlic powder, salt, and pepper. Mix well to create a marinade.
➢ Add the cauliflower florets to the bowl and toss until they are evenly coated with the marinade.
➢ Spread the cauliflower florets in a single layer on the prepared baking sheet.
➢ Roast in the preheated oven for about 20-25 minutes, or until the cauliflower is tender and lightly browned, stirring halfway through.

- ➤ Remove from the oven and let the curry roasted cauliflower cool slightly before serving.
- ➤ Garnish with fresh cilantro, if desired.

Nutritional Values:

Please note that these values are approximate and may vary based on specific ingredients used and serving size.

Per serving (1/4 of the recipe):

Calories: 100
Total Fat: 7g
Saturated Fat: 1g
Total Carbohydrates: 7g (Net: 4g)
Fiber: 3g
Protein: 3g

Health Benefits:

Cauliflower: Cauliflower is a low-carb vegetable that is rich in vitamins C and K. It also contains antioxidants and fiber, which contribute to overall health and digestion.

Curry Powder and Spices: The combination of curry powder, paprika, turmeric, and cumin not only adds flavor but also provides health benefits. These spices are known for their anti-inflammatory and antioxidant properties.

How it Helps in Keto:

Curry roasted cauliflower is low in net carbs and provides a good amount of fiber and healthy fats. It can be enjoyed as a side dish or as a main course when paired with a protein source.

Best Time of the Day to Eat:

Curry roasted cauliflower can be enjoyed as a side dish or main course for lunch or dinner. It pairs well with grilled meats or can be incorporated into a keto-friendly Buddha bowl. As always, balance it with other meals to meet your daily macronutrient and calorie goals.

60 Keto Roasted Cabbage

Roasted cabbage is a simple and delicious dish that can be enjoyed on a keto diet. It's easy to prepare and makes a great side dish. Here's how you can make it:

Ingredients:

1 small head of Cabbage
2 tablespoons of Olive Oil
Salt and Pepper to taste
Optional seasonings: Garlic powder, Onion powder, Paprika, etc.

Instructions:

➤ Preheat your oven to 200°C (400°F) and line a baking sheet with parchment paper.
➤ Remove any loose outer leaves from the cabbage and cut it into wedges, keeping the core intact.
➤ Place the cabbage wedges on the prepared baking sheet and drizzle them with olive oil.
➤ Sprinkle salt, pepper, and any optional seasonings of your choice over the cabbage wedges.
➤ Rub the oil and seasonings evenly onto the cabbage wedges, making sure they are well coated.
➤ Roast in the preheated oven for about 25-30 minutes, or until the cabbage is tender and lightly browned, flipping the wedges once halfway through.
➤ Remove from the oven and let the roasted cabbage cool slightly before serving.

Nutritional Values:

Please note that these values are approximate and may vary based on specific ingredients used and serving size.

Per serving (1/4 of the cabbage):

Calories: 70
Total Fat: 5g
Saturated Fat: 1g
Total Carbohydrates: 6g (Net: 4g)
Fiber: 2g
Protein: 2g

Health Benefits:

Cabbage: Cabbage is a cruciferous vegetable that is low in calories and carbohydrates. It is a good source of vitamins C and K, as well as dietary fiber.

Olive Oil: Olive oil provides healthy monounsaturated fats, which are associated with various health benefits, including heart health and reduced inflammation.

How it Helps in Keto:

Roasted cabbage is low in net carbs and provides a moderate amount of healthy fats. It can be enjoyed as a side dish or used as a base for other keto recipes.

Best Time of the Day to Eat:

Roasted cabbage can be enjoyed as a side dish for lunch or dinner. It pairs well with grilled meats or can be incorporated into keto-friendly salads or wraps. As always, balance it with other meals to meet your daily macronutrient and calorie goals.

61 Keto Brussels Sprouts with Creamy Mustard Sauce

Brussels sprouts with creamy mustard sauce is a flavorful and satisfying side dish that is perfect for a keto diet. Here's how you can make it:

Ingredients:

2 cups of Brussels Sprouts, halved
2 tablespoons of Olive Oil
Salt and Pepper to taste
1/4 cup of Heavy Cream
1 tablespoon of Dijon Mustard
1 tablespoon of Lemon Juice
Optional garnish: Chopped fresh parsley

Instructions:

➢ Preheat your oven to 200°C (400°F) and line a baking sheet with parchment paper.
➢ In a bowl, toss the halved Brussels sprouts with olive oil, salt, and pepper until well coated.
➢ Spread the Brussels sprouts in a single layer on the prepared baking sheet.
➢ Roast in the preheated oven for about 20-25 minutes, or until the Brussels sprouts are tender and lightly browned, flipping them once halfway through.
➢ While the Brussels sprouts are roasting, prepare the creamy mustard sauce. In a small saucepan, heat the heavy cream over low heat until warm.
➢ Stir in the Dijon mustard and lemon juice. Continue stirring until the sauce is well combined and slightly thickened.

- ➤ Remove the roasted Brussels sprouts from the oven and drizzle the creamy mustard sauce over them.
- ➤ Toss the Brussels sprouts in the sauce until evenly coated.
- ➤ Garnish with chopped fresh parsley, if desired.

Nutritional Values:

Please note that these values are approximate and may vary based on specific ingredients used and serving size.

Per serving (1/4 of the recipe):

Calories: 120
Total Fat: 10g
Saturated Fat: 4g
Total Carbohydrates: 6g (Net: 4g)
Fiber: 2g
Protein: 2g

Health Benefits:

Brussels Sprouts: Brussels sprouts are low in calories and carbohydrates while being rich in fiber, vitamins C and K, and antioxidants.

Olive Oil: Olive oil provides healthy monounsaturated fats, which have been linked to various health benefits, including heart health and reduced inflammation.

Dijon Mustard: Dijon mustard is low in calories and adds a tangy flavor to the dish. It contains antioxidants and can aid in digestion.

How it Helps in Keto:

Brussels sprouts with creamy mustard sauce is low in net carbs and provides a moderate amount of healthy fats. It's a great option for adding variety and flavor to your keto meals.

Best Time of the Day to Eat:

Brussels sprouts with creamy mustard sauce can be enjoyed as a side dish for lunch or dinner. It pairs well with a variety of protein sources, such as grilled chicken or salmon. As always, balance it with other meals to meet your daily macronutrient and calorie goals.

62 Keto Mushroom and Spinach Saute

Mushroom and spinach sauté is a quick and flavorful dish that is perfect for a keto diet. It combines two nutrient-rich ingredients to create a delicious side dish or a light main course. Here's how you can make it:

Ingredients:

2 cups of Mushrooms, sliced
2 cups of Fresh Spinach
2 cloves of Garlic, minced
2 tablespoons of Olive Oil
Salt and Pepper to taste
Optional seasonings: Red pepper flakes, Italian seasoning, etc.

Instructions:

- ➤ Heat the olive oil in a large skillet over medium heat.
- ➤ Add the minced garlic to the skillet and sauté for about 30 seconds until fragrant.
- ➤ Add the sliced mushrooms to the skillet and cook for about 5 minutes, stirring occasionally, until they release their moisture and start to brown.
- ➤ Add the fresh spinach to the skillet and cook for an additional 2-3 minutes until wilted.
- ➤ Season the mushroom and spinach mixture with salt, pepper, and any optional seasonings of your choice. Toss everything together until well combined.
- ➤ Remove from heat and serve hot.

Nutritional Values:

Please note that these values are approximate and may vary based on specific ingredients used and serving size.

Per serving (1/4 of the recipe):

Calories: 90
Total Fat: 7g
Saturated Fat: 1g
Total Carbohydrates: 5g (Net: 3g)
Fiber: 2g
Protein: 3g

Health Benefits:

Mushrooms: Mushrooms are low in calories and carbohydrates while being a good source of vitamins, minerals, and antioxidants. They are also a natural source of umami flavor.
Spinach: Spinach is packed with vitamins A, C, and K, as well as minerals like iron and magnesium. It's also low in calories and carbohydrates.

How it Helps in Keto:

Mushroom and spinach sauté is low in net carbs and provides a good amount of healthy fats and fiber. It's a great option for incorporating nutrient-dense vegetables into your keto diet.

Best Time of the Day to Eat:

You can enjoy mushroom and spinach sauté as a side dish for lunch or dinner. It pairs well with grilled meats or can be used as a topping for keto-friendly pizzas or omelets. As always, balance it with other meals to meet your daily macronutrient and calorie goals.

63Keto Zucchini Noodles with Creamy Avocado Pesto

Zucchini noodles with creamy avocado pesto is a delicious and nutritious dish that replaces traditional pasta with low-carb zucchini noodles. It's a perfect keto-friendly alternative that is packed with flavor and healthy fats. Here's how you can make it:

Ingredients:

For the zucchini noodles:

3 medium Zucchini
1 tablespoon of Olive Oil
Salt and Pepper to taste
For the creamy avocado pesto:

2 ripe Avocados
1 cup of Fresh Basil leaves
1/4 cup of Pine Nuts or Walnuts
2 cloves of Garlic
Juice of 1 Lemon
2 tablespoons of Olive Oil
Salt and Pepper to taste
Optional garnish: Grated Parmesan cheese, Red pepper flakes, Fresh basil leaves

Instructions:

For the zucchini noodles:

> Using a spiralizer or a vegetable peeler, create zucchini noodles from the zucchini. If using a vegetable peeler,

continue peeling the zucchini until you reach the seeded core.

➢ Heat olive oil in a large skillet over medium heat.
➢ Add the zucchini noodles to the skillet and sauté for about 3-5 minutes until they are tender but still slightly crisp.
➢ Season with salt and pepper to taste. Remove from heat and set aside.

For the creamy avocado pesto:

➢ In a food processor or blender, combine the ripe avocados, basil leaves, pine nuts or walnuts, garlic, lemon juice, olive oil, salt, and pepper.
➢ Process or blend until smooth and creamy. If the pesto is too thick, you can add a tablespoon of water at a time until you reach your desired consistency.
➢ Taste and adjust the seasoning if needed.

To serve:

➢ Toss the zucchini noodles with the creamy avocado pesto until well coated.
➢ Garnish with grated Parmesan cheese, red pepper flakes, and fresh basil leaves, if desired.
➢ Serve immediately.

Nutritional Values:

Please note that these values are approximate and may vary based on specific ingredients used and serving size.

Per serving (1/4 of the recipe):

Calories: 290
Total Fat: 25g

Saturated Fat: 4g
Total Carbohydrates: 15g (Net: 8g)
Fiber: 7g
Protein: 6g

Health Benefits:

Zucchini: Zucchini is a low-carb vegetable that is rich in vitamins, minerals, and dietary fiber. It adds bulk to the dish without adding excess carbohydrates.

Avocado: Avocado is a nutrient-dense fruit that provides heart-healthy monounsaturated fats, fiber, and various vitamins and minerals.

How it Helps in Keto:

Zucchini noodles with creamy avocado pesto is a keto-friendly alternative to traditional pasta dishes. It's low in net carbs and provides a good amount of healthy fats and fiber. This dish allows you to enjoy a satisfying meal while staying in ketosis.

Best Time of the Day to Eat:

You can enjoy zucchini noodles with creamy avocado pesto as a main course for lunch or dinner. It can be served on its own or paired with grilled chicken or shrimp for added protein. As always, balance it with other meals to meet your daily macronutrient and calorie goals.

64 Keto Spicy Roasted Peanuts

Spicy roasted peanuts are a crunchy and flavorful snack that can be enjoyed on a keto diet. They are perfect for satisfying your cravings and providing a dose of healthy fats. Here's how you can make them:

Ingredients:

2 cups of Raw Peanuts
1 tablespoon of Olive Oil
1 teaspoon of Smoked Paprika
1/2 teaspoon of Cayenne Pepper (adjust to your spice preference)
1/2 teaspoon of Garlic Powder
1/2 teaspoon of Onion Powder
1/2 teaspoon of Salt

Instructions:

➢ Preheat your oven to 160°C (325°F) and line a baking sheet with parchment paper.
➢ In a bowl, toss the raw peanuts with olive oil until well coated.
➢ In a separate small bowl, mix together the smoked paprika, cayenne pepper, garlic powder, onion powder, and salt.
➢ Sprinkle the spice mixture over the peanuts and toss until the peanuts are evenly coated with the spices.
➢ Spread the seasoned peanuts in a single layer on the prepared baking sheet.
➢ Roast in the preheated oven for about 15-20 minutes, or until the peanuts are golden brown and fragrant, stirring them halfway through.

➢ Remove from the oven and let the spicy roasted peanuts cool completely before serving.

Nutritional Values:

Please note that these values are approximate and may vary based on specific ingredients used and serving size.

Per serving (1/4 cup):

Calories: 170
Total Fat: 15g
Saturated Fat: 2g
Total Carbohydrates: 5g (Net: 3g)
Fiber: 2g
Protein: 7g

Health Benefits:

Peanuts: Peanuts are a good source of healthy fats, protein, and fiber. They also contain various vitamins and minerals, including vitamin E and magnesium.

How it Helps in Keto:

Spicy roasted peanuts are low in net carbs and provide a good amount of healthy fats and protein. They make a satisfying keto-friendly snack that can help curb hunger and keep you in ketosis.

Best Time of the Day to Eat:

Spicy roasted peanuts can be enjoyed as a snack throughout the day. They are great for on-the-go or as a crunchy addition to your keto trail mix. Just be mindful of portion sizes to stay within your daily calorie goals.

65 Keto Paneer Jalfrezi

Paneer jalfrezi is a delicious and spicy Indian dish that features paneer (Indian cottage cheese) and a variety of colorful vegetables. It's a popular vegetarian option that can be enjoyed on a keto diet. Here's how you can make it:

Ingredients:

200 grams of Paneer, cut into cubes
1 Green Bell Pepper, thinly sliced
1 Red Bell Pepper, thinly sliced
1 Yellow Bell Pepper, thinly sliced
1 Onion, thinly sliced
2 Tomatoes, chopped
2 Green Chilies, slit lengthwise
2 tablespoons of Ghee or Coconut Oil
1 teaspoon of Cumin Seeds
1 teaspoon of Ginger-Garlic Paste
1 teaspoon of Turmeric Powder
1 teaspoon of Kashmiri Red Chili Powder (adjust to your spice preference)
1 teaspoon of Garam Masala
Salt to taste
Fresh Cilantro for garnish

Instructions:

➢ Heat ghee or coconut oil in a large skillet or wok over medium heat.
➢ Add the cumin seeds and let them splutter.
➢ Add the thinly sliced onions and sauté until they turn golden brown.

- ➢ Add the ginger-garlic paste and green chilies. Sauté for a minute until fragrant.
- ➢ Add the chopped tomatoes and cook until they become soft and mushy.
- ➢ Add the turmeric powder, red chili powder, and salt. Mix well.
- ➢ Add the thinly sliced bell peppers and cook for about 3-4 minutes until they are slightly tender but still retain their crunch.
- ➢ Add the paneer cubes and garam masala. Gently toss everything together until the paneer is coated with the spices.
- ➢ Cook for an additional 2-3 minutes until the paneer is heated through.
- ➢ Remove from heat and garnish with fresh cilantro.

Nutritional Values:

Please note that these values are approximate and may vary based on specific ingredients used and serving size.

Per serving (1/4 of the recipe):

Calories: 280
Total Fat: 21g
Saturated Fat: 12g
Total Carbohydrates: 9g (Net: 6g)
Fiber: 3g
Protein: 15g

Health Benefits:

Paneer: Paneer is a good source of protein and calcium, making it beneficial for bone health and muscle development.

Bell Peppers: Bell peppers are rich in vitamins A and C, as well as antioxidants. They can support immune function and contribute to overall health.

How it Helps in Keto:

Paneer jalfrezi is low in net carbs and provides a good amount of protein and healthy fats. It's a satisfying and flavorful dish that can be enjoyed as a main course for lunch or dinner.

Best Time of the Day to Eat:

Paneer jalfrezi can be enjoyed as a main course for lunch or dinner. It can be served with cauliflower rice or keto-friendly flatbreads. As always, balance it with other meals to meet your daily macronutrient and calorie goals.

66 Keto Spiced Cauliflower Rice

Spiced cauliflower rice is a low-carb and flavorful alternative to traditional rice. It's easy to make and can be used as a base for various keto-friendly dishes. Here's how you can make it:

Ingredients:

1 medium head of Cauliflower
2 tablespoons of Olive Oil or Ghee
1/2 teaspoon of Cumin Seeds
1/2 teaspoon of Turmeric Powder
1/2 teaspoon of Paprika
Salt and Pepper to taste
Optional add-ins: Minced garlic, Chopped onions, Diced bell peppers, etc.

Instructions:

- Cut the cauliflower into florets and discard the tough core.
- Place the cauliflower florets in a food processor and pulse until they reach a rice-like consistency. Be careful not to over-process, as it can turn into a mushy texture.
- Heat olive oil or ghee in a large skillet over medium heat.
- Add the cumin seeds and let them splutter.
- If using, add minced garlic, chopped onions, or any other optional add-ins to the skillet. Sauté until the onions are translucent and the vegetables are tender.
- Add the riced cauliflower to the skillet and toss to combine with the spices and vegetables.
- Season with turmeric powder, paprika, salt, and pepper. Mix well to evenly distribute the spices.

➤ Cook for about 5-7 minutes, stirring occasionally, until the cauliflower rice is tender but still retains its texture. Be careful not to overcook, as it can become mushy.
➤ Remove from heat and serve hot.

Nutritional Values:

Please note that these values are approximate and may vary based on specific ingredients used and serving size.

Per serving (1/4 of the recipe):

Calories: 90
Total Fat: 7g
Saturated Fat: 1g
Total Carbohydrates: 6g (Net: 3g)
Fiber: 3g
Protein: 3g

Health Benefits:

Cauliflower: Cauliflower is a low-carb vegetable that is rich in vitamins C and K. It also contains antioxidants and fiber, which contribute to overall health and digestion.

How it Helps in Keto:

Spiced cauliflower rice is low in net carbs and provides a good amount of fiber and healthy fats. It can be used as a base for various keto-friendly dishes, such as stir-fries, fried rice alternatives, or as a side dish.

Best Time of the Day to Eat:

Spiced cauliflower rice can be enjoyed as a side dish or used as a base for main courses for lunch or dinner. It pairs well with various protein sources and can be incorporated into a variety of keto recipes. As always, balance it with other meals to meet your daily macronutrient and calorie goals.

67 Keto Broccoli and Cheese Stuffed Bell Peppers

Broccoli and cheese stuffed bell peppers are a delicious and nutritious keto-friendly dish that combines the flavors of roasted bell peppers, tender broccoli, and melty cheese. Here's how you can make them:

Ingredients:

4 large Bell Peppers (any color)
2 cups of Broccoli florets, steamed or blanched
1 cup of Shredded Cheddar Cheese (or any cheese of your choice)
1/4 cup of Heavy Cream
2 tablespoons of Butter
1/2 teaspoon of Garlic Powder
Salt and Pepper to taste
Optional garnish: Chopped fresh parsley

Instructions:

➤ Preheat your oven to 200°C (400°F) and line a baking dish with parchment paper.
➤ Cut the bell peppers in half lengthwise and remove the seeds and membranes.
➤ In a large pot of boiling water, blanch the bell pepper halves for 2-3 minutes to slightly soften them. Drain and set aside.
➤ In a mixing bowl, combine the steamed or blanched broccoli florets, shredded cheddar cheese, heavy cream, butter, garlic powder, salt, and pepper. Mix well until everything is evenly combined.

- ➤ Fill each bell pepper half with the broccoli and cheese mixture, pressing it down gently to fill the cavity.
- ➤ Place the stuffed bell peppers in the prepared baking dish and cover with foil.
- ➤ Bake in the preheated oven for about 20-25 minutes, or until the bell peppers are tender and the cheese is melted and bubbly.
- ➤ Remove from the oven and let them cool for a few minutes before serving.
- ➤ Garnish with chopped fresh parsley, if desired.

Nutritional Values:

Please note that these values are approximate and may vary based on specific ingredients used and serving size.

Per serving (1 stuffed bell pepper half):

Calories: 170
Total Fat: 14g
Saturated Fat: 9g
Total Carbohydrates: 7g (Net: 4g)
Fiber: 3g
Protein: 7g

Health Benefits:

Bell Peppers: Bell peppers are low in calories and rich in vitamins A and C. They also provide antioxidants and dietary fiber.
Broccoli: Broccoli is a nutrient-dense vegetable that is high in vitamins C and K, as well as folate and fiber. It also contains various antioxidants.

How it Helps in Keto:

Broccoli and cheese stuffed bell peppers are low in net carbs and provide a good amount of healthy fats, fiber, and protein. They make a satisfying keto-friendly meal or side dish.

Best Time of the Day to Eat:

Broccoli and cheese stuffed bell peppers can be enjoyed as a main course for lunch or dinner. They pair well with a side salad or can be served with grilled chicken or fish for added protein. As always, balance it with other meals to meet your daily macronutrient and calorie goals.

68 Keto Spiced Pumpkin Soup with Coconut Milk

Keto spiced pumpkin soup with coconut milk is a warm and comforting dish that is perfect for the fall season. It combines the flavors of pumpkin, aromatic spices, and creamy coconut milk. Here's how you can make it:

Ingredients:

2 cups of Pumpkin Puree (canned or homemade)
1 can (13.5 oz) of Coconut Milk (full-fat)
1 small Onion, diced
2 cloves of Garlic, minced
1 teaspoon of Ginger, grated
1 teaspoon of Ground Cumin
1/2 teaspoon of Ground Coriander
1/2 teaspoon of Ground Cinnamon
1/4 teaspoon of Ground Nutmeg
1/4 teaspoon of Cayenne Pepper (adjust to your spice preference)
2 cups of Vegetable Broth
2 tablespoons of Olive Oil or Coconut Oil
Salt and Pepper to taste
Optional garnish: Fresh cilantro or pumpkin seeds

Instructions:

➢ Heat olive oil or coconut oil in a large pot or Dutch oven over medium heat.
➢ Add the diced onion and sauté until it becomes translucent.
➢ Add the minced garlic and grated ginger. Sauté for a minute until fragrant.

- ➤ Add the ground cumin, ground coriander, ground cinnamon, ground nutmeg, and cayenne pepper. Stir well to toast the spices for about a minute.
- ➤ Add the pumpkin puree, coconut milk, and vegetable broth to the pot. Stir until everything is well combined.
- ➤ Season with salt and pepper to taste.
- ➤ Bring the soup to a simmer and let it cook for about 10-15 minutes to allow the flavors to meld together.
- ➤ Remove the pot from heat and use an immersion blender or a countertop blender to puree the soup until smooth and creamy.
- ➤ If needed, return the soup to the heat and warm it through.
- ➤ Ladle the soup into bowls and garnish with fresh cilantro or pumpkin seeds, if desired.

Nutritional Values:

Please note that these values are approximate and may vary based on specific ingredients used and serving size.

Per serving (1/4 of the recipe):

Calories: 230
Total Fat: 20g
Saturated Fat: 16g
Total Carbohydrates: 9g (Net: 6g)
Fiber: 3g
Protein: 3g

Health Benefits:

Pumpkin: Pumpkin is low in calories and rich in vitamins A and C. It's also a good source of fiber and antioxidants.

Coconut Milk: Coconut milk provides healthy fats and can contribute to a feeling of fullness. It also adds creaminess to the soup.

How it Helps in Keto:

Keto spiced pumpkin soup with coconut milk is low in net carbs and provides a good amount of healthy fats. It's a flavorful and satisfying option for a keto-friendly soup.

Best Time of the Day to Eat:

Keto spiced pumpkin soup with coconut milk can be enjoyed as a starter or a light meal for lunch or dinner. It pairs well with a side salad or a keto-friendly bread roll. As always, balance it with other meals to meet your daily macronutrient and calorie goals.

69 Keto Almond Flour Roti

Keto almond flour roti is a versatile and grain-free alternative to traditional wheat-based roti. It's soft, pliable, and can be used to wrap various fillings or served as a side with curries or stews. Here's how you can make it:

Ingredients:

1 cup of Almond Flour
2 tablespoons of Ground Flaxseed
1/4 teaspoon of Xanthan Gum (optional, helps with binding)
1/4 teaspoon of Salt
1/2 cup of Hot Water
Ghee or Coconut Oil for greasing

Instructions:

➤ In a mixing bowl, combine the almond flour, ground flaxseed, xanthan gum (if using), and salt. Mix well to combine.

➤ Gradually add the hot water to the dry ingredients while stirring continuously. Continue to mix until a dough forms.

➤ Knead the dough for a few minutes until it becomes smooth and pliable. If the dough feels too dry, add a little more hot water, one tablespoon at a time. If it feels too sticky, add a little more almond flour.

➤ Divide the dough into equal-sized balls. You should get around 4-6 balls, depending on the size of the roti you prefer.

➤ Place a ball of dough between two sheets of parchment paper. Using a rolling pin, roll out the dough into a thin, round roti.

- ➤ Heat a skillet or tawa over medium-high heat.
- ➤ Carefully transfer the rolled-out roti onto the hot skillet. Cook for about 1-2 minutes on one side, or until it starts to bubble and brown spots appear.
- ➤ Flip the roti and cook for another 1-2 minutes on the other side.
- ➤ Remove from the skillet and brush the roti with ghee or coconut oil.
- ➤ Repeat the process with the remaining dough balls.
- ➤ Serve the almond flour roti warm as a wrap for fillings or as a side with curries or stews.

Nutritional Values:

Please note that these values are approximate and may vary based on specific ingredients used and serving size.

Per serving (1 roti, based on 4 servings):

Calories: 190
Total Fat: 17g
Saturated Fat: 2g
Total Carbohydrates: 7g (Net: 3g)
Fiber: 4g
Protein: 7g
Health Benefits:

Almond Flour: Almond flour is low in carbs and rich in healthy fats, protein, and fiber. It also provides vitamin E and magnesium.
Ground Flaxseed: Ground flaxseed is a good source of omega-3 fatty acids, fiber, and lignans, which are beneficial for heart health.

How it Helps in Keto:

Keto almond flour roti is low in net carbs and provides a good amount of healthy fats and fiber. It's a great option for those following a keto diet and looking for a grain-free alternative to traditional roti.

Best Time of the Day to Eat:

Keto almond flour roti can be enjoyed as a meal component at any time of the day. It can be used as a wrap for breakfast, lunch, or dinner fillings, or served as a side with keto-friendly curries or stews.

70 Keto Chilled Cucumber Soup

Keto chilled cucumber soup is a refreshing and light dish that is perfect for hot summer days. It's made with fresh cucumbers, herbs, and a creamy base. Here's how you can make it:

Ingredients:

4 large Cucumbers, peeled and seeded
1 cup of Greek Yogurt (full-fat)
1/4 cup of Fresh Mint Leaves
1/4 cup of Fresh Dill
2 tablespoons of Fresh Lemon Juice
2 cloves of Garlic
2 tablespoons of Olive Oil
Salt and Pepper to taste
Optional garnish: Chopped fresh herbs, sliced cucumber

Instructions:

- ➤ Slice the peeled and seeded cucumbers into chunks and place them in a blender or food processor.
- ➤ Add the Greek yogurt, fresh mint leaves, fresh dill, fresh lemon juice, garlic cloves, olive oil, salt, and pepper to the blender.
- ➤ Blend until smooth and creamy. If needed, add a little water to achieve the desired consistency.
- ➤ Taste and adjust the seasoning if necessary.
- ➤ Transfer the soup to a container and refrigerate for at least 1 hour to chill and allow the flavors to meld together.
- ➤ Serve the chilled cucumber soup in bowls or glasses.
- ➤ Garnish with chopped fresh herbs and sliced cucumber, if desired.

Nutritional Values:

Please note that these values are approximate and may vary based on specific ingredients used and serving size.

Per serving (1/4 of the recipe):

Calories: 120
Total Fat: 8g
Saturated Fat: 2g
Total Carbohydrates: 8g (Net: 4g)
Fiber: 4g
Protein: 6g

Health Benefits:

Cucumber: Cucumbers are low in calories and high in water content, making them hydrating. They also provide vitamins K and C, as well as antioxidants.

Greek Yogurt: Greek yogurt is rich in protein, calcium, and probiotics, which can support gut health.

How it Helps in Keto:

Keto chilled cucumber soup is low in net carbs and provides a good amount of protein and healthy fats from the Greek yogurt. It's a refreshing and hydrating option for a keto-friendly soup.

Best Time of the Day to Eat:

Keto chilled cucumber soup is best enjoyed as a light meal or a refreshing snack during hot summer days. It can be served as an appetizer or enjoyed as a light lunch or dinner option.

71 Keto Baked Cauliflower Tots

Keto baked cauliflower tots are a delicious and healthier alternative to traditional potato tots. They are made with cauliflower as the base, mixed with cheese and seasonings, and baked to perfection. Here's how you can make them:

Ingredients:

1 medium head of Cauliflower, cut into florets
1/2 cup of Shredded Cheddar Cheese
1/4 cup of Grated Parmesan Cheese
1/4 cup of Almond Flour
1 teaspoon of Garlic Powder
1/2 teaspoon of Onion Powder
1/2 teaspoon of Paprika
1/4 teaspoon of Salt
1/4 teaspoon of Black Pepper
1 large Egg, beaten
Optional add-ins: Chopped fresh herbs, minced garlic, diced onions, etc.

Instructions:

- ➤ Preheat your oven to 200°C (400°F) and line a baking sheet with parchment paper.
- ➤ Steam or blanch the cauliflower florets until they are fork-tender. Drain well and let them cool slightly.
- ➤ Place the cooked cauliflower florets in a clean kitchen towel or cheesecloth. Squeeze out any excess moisture to ensure the tots hold their shape.

- ➢ Transfer the cauliflower to a food processor and pulse a few times until it resembles rice-like grains. Be careful not to overprocess, as it can become mushy.
- ➢ In a mixing bowl, combine the cauliflower rice, shredded cheddar cheese, grated Parmesan cheese, almond flour, garlic powder, onion powder, paprika, salt, and black pepper. Mix well to combine.
- ➢ Add the beaten egg to the cauliflower mixture and mix until everything is evenly incorporated. The mixture should be sticky enough to hold together.
- ➢ Take a small portion of the mixture and shape it into a tot-like shape. Place it on the prepared baking sheet. Repeat until all the mixture is used, spacing the tots evenly on the baking sheet.
- ➢ Bake in the preheated oven for about 20-25 minutes, or until the tots are golden brown and crispy on the outside.
- ➢ Remove from the oven and let them cool for a few minutes before serving.

Nutritional Values:

Please note that these values are approximate and may vary based on specific ingredients used and serving size.

Per serving (about 4 tots):

Calories: 100
Total Fat: 7g
Saturated Fat: 3g
Total Carbohydrates: 5g (Net: 3g)
Fiber: 2g
Protein: 6g
Health Benefits:

Cauliflower: Cauliflower is a low-carb vegetable that is rich in vitamins C and K. It's also a good source of fiber and antioxidants.

Cheddar Cheese: Cheddar cheese provides protein, calcium, and vitamin K2. It can also contribute to a feeling of satiety.

How it Helps in Keto:

Keto baked cauliflower tots are low in net carbs and provide a good amount of healthy fats, fiber, and protein. They make a satisfying and flavorful alternative to traditional potato tots.

Best Time of the Day to Eat:

Keto baked cauliflower tots can be enjoyed as a snack, appetizer, or side dish at any time of the day. They pair well with keto-friendly dips or sauces. As always, balance it with other meals to meet your daily macronutrient and calorie goals.

72 Keto Avocado Egg Salad

Keto avocado egg salad is a flavorful and nutritious dish that combines creamy avocados with protein-rich eggs. It's easy to make and can be enjoyed as a filling and satisfying meal. Here's how you can make it:

Ingredients:

4 hard-boiled Eggs, peeled and chopped
2 ripe Avocados, pitted and mashed
2 tablespoons of Mayonnaise (preferably avocado oil-based)
1 tablespoon of Lemon Juice
2 tablespoons of chopped Fresh Parsley
1 tablespoon of chopped Fresh Chives (optional)
Salt and Pepper to taste

Instructions:

➢ In a mixing bowl, combine the chopped hard-boiled eggs, mashed avocados, mayonnaise, lemon juice, chopped parsley, and chopped chives (if using). Mix well to combine.

➢ Season with salt and pepper to taste. Adjust the amount of lemon juice, mayo, or seasonings based on your preference.

➢ Gently fold the ingredients together until the egg salad is evenly mixed.

➢ Cover the bowl and refrigerate for at least 30 minutes to allow the flavors to meld together.

➢ Serve the keto avocado egg salad on its own, as a sandwich filling, or as a topping for salads or low-carb wraps.

Nutritional Values:

Please note that these values are approximate and may vary based on specific ingredients used and serving size.

Per serving (about 1/2 cup):

Calories: 230
Total Fat: 20g
Saturated Fat: 4g
Total Carbohydrates: 5g (Net: 2g)
Fiber: 3g
Protein: 8g

Health Benefits:

Avocado: Avocado is a nutrient-dense fruit that is high in healthy fats, fiber, and vitamins. It also provides potassium and antioxidants.

Eggs: Eggs are an excellent source of protein and provide essential vitamins and minerals such as vitamin D, vitamin B12, and selenium.

How it Helps in Keto:

Keto avocado egg salad is low in net carbs and provides a good amount of healthy fats and protein. It makes a satisfying and filling option for a keto-friendly meal.

Best Time of the Day to Eat:

Keto avocado egg salad can be enjoyed as a meal for breakfast, lunch, or dinner. It's versatile and can be served in various ways, such as on lettuce wraps, with keto-friendly bread, or alongside fresh vegetables. As always, balance it with other meals to meet your daily macronutrient and calorie goals.

73 Keto Spinach and Artichoke Dip

Keto spinach and artichoke dip is a creamy and flavorful appetizer that is perfect for gatherings or as a snack. It's made with a combination of spinach, artichoke hearts, and cheese. Here's how you can make it:

Ingredients:

8 ounces of Frozen Spinach, thawed and drained
1 can (14 ounces) of Artichoke Hearts, drained and chopped
1/2 cup of Mayonnaise (preferably avocado oil-based)
1/2 cup of Sour Cream (full-fat)
1/2 cup of Cream Cheese (full-fat), softened
1/4 cup of Grated Parmesan Cheese
1/4 cup of Shredded Mozzarella Cheese
2 cloves of Garlic, minced
1/2 teaspoon of Onion Powder
1/2 teaspoon of Garlic Powder
Salt and Pepper to taste

Instructions:

- ➢ Preheat your oven to 180°C (350°F).
- ➢ In a mixing bowl, combine the thawed and drained spinach, chopped artichoke hearts, mayonnaise, sour cream, cream cheese, grated Parmesan cheese, shredded mozzarella cheese, minced garlic, onion powder, garlic powder, salt, and pepper. Mix well to combine.
- ➢ Transfer the mixture to a baking dish or cast-iron skillet.
- ➢ Bake in the preheated oven for about 20-25 minutes, or until the top is golden brown and bubbling.

- ➢ Remove from the oven and let it cool for a few minutes before serving.
- ➢ Serve the keto spinach and artichoke dip with low-carb vegetables, keto-friendly crackers

Nutritional Values:

Please note that these values are approximate and may vary based on specific ingredients used and serving size.

Per serving (about 1/4 cup):

Calories: 180
Total Fat: 16g
Saturated Fat: 6g
Total Carbohydrates: 5g (Net: 3g)
Fiber: 2g
Protein: 5g

Health Benefits:

Spinach: Spinach is rich in vitamins A, C, and K, as well as iron and antioxidants. It provides essential nutrients and supports overall health.

Artichoke Hearts: Artichoke hearts are low in calories and high in fiber, vitamins, and minerals. They also contain antioxidants that can benefit health.

How it Helps in Keto:

Keto spinach and artichoke dip is low in net carbs and provides a good amount of healthy fats and fiber. It makes a delicious and satisfying option for a keto-friendly appetizer or snack.

Best Time of the Day to Eat:

Keto spinach and artichoke dip can be enjoyed as a snack or appetizer. It's great for gatherings, parties, or when you're craving a savory and creamy dip. Enjoy it with keto-friendly accompaniments or as a topping for low-carb bread or crackers.

74 Keto Tomato and Basil Salad

Keto tomato and basil salad is a simple and refreshing dish that showcases the flavors of ripe tomatoes and fragrant basil. It's light, vibrant, and pairs well with a variety of main courses. Here's how you can make it:

Ingredients:

4 medium-sized Tomatoes, sliced
1/4 cup of Fresh Basil Leaves, torn or chopped
2 tablespoons of Extra Virgin Olive Oil
1 tablespoon of Balsamic Vinegar (optional)
Salt and Pepper to taste

Instructions:

➢ Arrange the tomato slices on a serving platter or individual plates.
➢ Sprinkle the torn or chopped basil leaves over the tomatoes.
➢ Drizzle the extra virgin olive oil and balsamic vinegar (if using) over the salad.
➢ Season with salt and pepper to taste.
➢ Gently toss the salad to ensure the flavors are evenly distributed.
➢ Let the salad sit at room temperature for a few minutes to allow the flavors to meld together before serving.

Nutritional Values:

Please note that these values are approximate and may vary based on specific ingredients used and serving size.

Per serving (1/2 of the recipe):

Calories: 110
Total Fat: 9g
Saturated Fat: 1g
Total Carbohydrates: 6g (Net: 4g)
Fiber: 2g
Protein: 1g

Health Benefits:

Tomatoes: Tomatoes are rich in lycopene, an antioxidant that has been linked to various health benefits. They are also a good source of vitamins C and K, potassium, and folate.

Basil: Basil is an aromatic herb that provides vitamins A, K, and C, as well as antioxidants. It adds a fresh and herbaceous flavor to dishes.

How it Helps in Keto:

Keto tomato and basil salad is low in net carbs and provides a moderate amount of healthy fats. It's a light and refreshing option that can be enjoyed as a side dish or incorporated into a larger meal.

Best Time of the Day to Eat:

Keto tomato and basil salad can be enjoyed as a side dish for any meal. It complements various cuisines and works well alongside grilled meats, seafood, or as part of a salad spread. Enjoy it when tomatoes are in season for the best flavor and taste.

75 Keto Cabbage Soup

Keto cabbage soup is a comforting and nourishing dish that is packed with vegetables and flavor. It's a great option for those looking for a low-carb and nutrient-dense soup. Here's how you can make it:

Ingredients:

2 tablespoons of Olive Oil or Avocado Oil
1 medium Onion, diced
2 cloves of Garlic, minced
4 cups of Vegetable Broth (or chicken broth if preferred)
4 cups of shredded Cabbage
2 medium Carrots, peeled and diced
2 stalks of Celery, diced
1 can (14 ounces) of Diced Tomatoes
1 teaspoon of Dried Thyme
1 teaspoon of Dried Oregano
Salt and Pepper to taste
Optional garnish: Fresh parsley or cilantro, grated Parmesan cheese

Instructions:

➢ In a large pot or Dutch oven, heat the olive oil or avocado oil over medium heat.
➢ Add the diced onion and minced garlic to the pot. Sauté until the onion becomes translucent and fragrant.
➢ Pour in the vegetable broth and bring it to a simmer.
➢ Add the shredded cabbage, diced carrots, diced celery, diced tomatoes (with their juices), dried thyme, dried oregano, salt, and pepper to the pot. Stir well to combine.

- ➢ Cover the pot and let the soup simmer for about 20-25 minutes, or until the vegetables are tender.
- ➢ Taste the soup and adjust the seasonings if necessary.
- ➢ Ladle the keto cabbage soup into bowls and garnish with fresh parsley or cilantro and grated Parmesan cheese, if desired.

Nutritional Values:

Please note that these values are approximate and may vary based on specific ingredients used and serving size.

Per serving (about 1 cup):

Calories: 90
Total Fat: 4g
Saturated Fat: 0.5g
Total Carbohydrates: 10g (Net: 7g)
Fiber: 3g
Protein: 2g

Health Benefits:

Cabbage: Cabbage is low in calories and high in fiber, vitamins C and K, and antioxidants. It's also known for its potential anti-inflammatory properties.

Carrots: Carrots are rich in beta-carotene, which converts to vitamin A in the body. They also provide fiber and antioxidants.

How it Helps in Keto:

Keto cabbage soup is low in net carbs and provides a good amount of fiber and nutrients from the vegetables. It's a satisfying and comforting option for a keto-friendly soup.

Best Time of the Day to Eat:

Keto cabbage soup can be enjoyed as a light meal or as a starter to a larger meal. It's versatile and can be enjoyed for lunch or dinner. Feel free to customize the recipe with additional protein, such as cooked chicken or ground meat, to make it more filling and suitable for any time of the day.

76 Keto Spiced Roasted Cauliflower

Keto spiced roasted cauliflower is a flavorful and nutritious side dish that brings out the natural sweetness and texture of cauliflower. It's seasoned with aromatic spices and roasted to perfection. Here's how you can make it:

Ingredients:

1 large head of Cauliflower, cut into florets

2 tablespoons of Olive Oil or Avocado Oil

1 teaspoon of Paprika

1/2 teaspoon of Ground Cumin

1/2 teaspoon of Ground Coriander

1/2 teaspoon of Garlic Powder

1/2 teaspoon of Onion Powder

1/4 teaspoon of Cayenne Pepper (optional for heat)

Salt and Pepper to taste

Fresh cilantro or parsley for garnish (optional)

Instructions:

➢ Preheat your oven to 200°C (400°F) and line a baking sheet with parchment paper.

➢ In a large mixing bowl, combine the cauliflower florets, olive oil or avocado oil, paprika, ground cumin, ground coriander, garlic powder, onion powder, cayenne pepper (if using), salt, and pepper. Toss well to coat the cauliflower evenly with the spices and oil.

➢ Spread the seasoned cauliflower florets in a single layer on the prepared baking sheet.

➢ Roast in the preheated oven for about 20-25 minutes, or until the cauliflower is golden brown and tender, with a slight crispness on the edges.

- ➤ Remove from the oven and let it cool for a few minutes. Garnish with fresh cilantro or parsley, if desired.
- ➤ Serve the keto spiced roasted cauliflower as a side dish or as part of a larger meal.

Nutritional Values:

Please note that these values are approximate and may vary based on specific ingredients used and serving size.

Per serving (about 1 cup):

Calories: 100
Total Fat: 7g
Saturated Fat: 1g
Total Carbohydrates: 7g (Net: 4g)
Fiber: 3g
Protein: 3g

Health Benefits:

Cauliflower: Cauliflower is a versatile vegetable that is low in calories and high in fiber, vitamins C and K, and antioxidants. It's also a good source of choline, which supports brain health.
Spices: The spices used in this recipe, such as paprika, cumin, coriander, and garlic powder, not only add flavor but also provide potential health benefits due to their antioxidant and anti-inflammatory properties.

How it Helps in Keto:

Keto spiced roasted cauliflower is low in net carbs and provides a good amount of fiber. It's a tasty and satisfying option to incorporate nutrient-dense vegetables into your keto diet.

Best Time of the Day to Eat:

Keto spiced roasted cauliflower can be enjoyed as a side dish for any meal. It complements various protein sources and can be part of a well-balanced lunch or dinner. Enjoy it hot from the oven or at room temperature as a snack or appetizer.

77 Keto Coconut and Almond Flour Flatbread

Keto coconut and almond flour flatbread is a delicious and versatile option that can be used as a low-carb bread substitute. It's gluten-free, grain-free, and easy to make. Here's how you can make it:

Ingredients:

1/2 cup of Coconut Flour
1/2 cup of Almond Flour
4 large Eggs
1/4 cup of Coconut Milk (full-fat)
2 tablespoons of Olive Oil or Melted Coconut Oil
1/2 teaspoon of Baking Powder
1/4 teaspoon of Salt

Instructions:

➢ Preheat your oven to 180°C (350°F) and line a baking sheet with parchment paper.
➢ In a mixing bowl, whisk together the coconut flour, almond flour, baking powder, and salt.
➢ In a separate bowl, whisk together the eggs, coconut milk, and olive oil or melted coconut oil.
➢ Add the wet ingredients to the dry ingredients and stir until well combined. The mixture will be thick.
➢ Let the mixture sit for a few minutes to allow the coconut flour to absorb the liquid. If the mixture becomes too thick, you can add a tablespoon of water or additional coconut milk.

- ➤ Divide the dough into 4 equal portions and shape each portion into a round flatbread shape, about 1/4 inch thick, on the prepared baking sheet.
- ➤ Bake in the preheated oven for about 12-15 minutes, or until the flatbreads are set and slightly golden around the edges.
- ➤ Remove from the oven and let them cool slightly before serving.

Nutritional Values:

Please note that these values are approximate and may vary based on specific ingredients used and serving size.

Per serving (1 flatbread):

Calories: 130
Total Fat: 10g
Saturated Fat: 3g
Total Carbohydrates: 6g (Net: 3g)
Fiber: 3g
Protein: 6g

Health Benefits:

Coconut Flour: Coconut flour is low in carbohydrates and high in fiber. It also contains healthy fats and provides some essential minerals.
Almond Flour: Almond flour is a nutrient-dense alternative to traditional flours. It's high in healthy fats, protein, and vitamin E.

How it Helps in Keto:

Keto coconut and almond flour flatbread is low in net carbs and provides a good amount of healthy fats and fiber. It can be used as a bread substitute in sandwiches, wraps, or as a base for keto-friendly pizza crust.

Best Time of the Day to Eat:

Keto coconut and almond flour flatbread can be enjoyed at any time of the day. It's a versatile option that can be used to create a variety of meals, such as breakfast sandwiches, lunch wraps, or as a side with dinner. Customize it with your favorite keto-friendly fillings and toppings.

78 Keto Grilled Vegetable Skewers

Keto grilled vegetable skewers are a colorful and flavorful dish that can be enjoyed as a side dish or a light meal. They are packed with nutrients and make a great addition to any barbecue or outdoor gathering. Here's how you can make them:

Ingredients:

Assorted Vegetables of your choice (e.g., Bell Peppers, Zucchini, Mushrooms, Cherry Tomatoes, Red Onion, Eggplant)
Olive Oil
Salt and Pepper to taste
Optional seasonings: Garlic powder, Italian herbs, Paprika, Lemon juice

Instructions:

➤ Soak wooden skewers in water for about 30 minutes to prevent them from burning on the grill.
➤ Prepare the vegetables by washing, trimming, and cutting them into bite-sized pieces.
➤ In a mixing bowl, drizzle the vegetables with olive oil and season with salt and pepper. Add any optional seasonings or herbs for additional flavor, if desired.
➤ Thread the vegetables onto the soaked skewers, alternating different vegetables for variety and color.
➤ Preheat your grill to medium heat.
➤ Place the vegetable skewers on the grill and cook for about 8-10 minutes, turning occasionally, until the vegetables are tender and lightly charred.
➤ Remove the skewers from the grill and let them cool slightly before serving.

Nutritional Values:

Please note that the nutritional values will vary depending on the types and amounts of vegetables used.

Health Benefits:

Assorted Vegetables: Grilled vegetables are rich in vitamins, minerals, and antioxidants. They provide essential nutrients and can support overall health and well-being.

How it Helps in Keto:

Keto grilled vegetable skewers are low in carbohydrates and provide fiber, vitamins, and minerals. They can be a satisfying and nutritious addition to a keto diet.

Best Time of the Day to Eat:

Keto grilled vegetable skewers can be enjoyed as a side dish for lunch or dinner. They pair well with grilled meats or can be served as a vegetarian option. Enjoy them as part of a keto-friendly barbecue or outdoor meal.

79 Keto Almond Flour Dosa

Keto almond flour dosa is a low-carb and grain-free alternative to traditional dosa, a popular Indian crepe. It's made with almond flour and other keto-friendly ingredients, offering a delicious and nutritious option. Here's how you can make it:

Ingredients:

1 cup of Almond Flour
2 tablespoons of Flaxseed Meal
2 tablespoons of Coconut Flour
1/4 cup of Plain Greek Yogurt
2 large Eggs
1/4 cup of Water (or more as needed)
1/2 teaspoon of Baking Powder
Salt to taste
Ghee or Coconut Oil for cooking

Instructions:

- ➤ In a mixing bowl, whisk together the almond flour, flaxseed meal, coconut flour, baking powder, and salt.
- ➤ In a separate bowl, beat the eggs and mix in the Greek yogurt.
- ➤ Combine the wet and dry ingredients, and gradually add water while whisking until you have a smooth and pourable batter. The consistency should be similar to pancake batter.
- ➤ Let the batter sit for about 10-15 minutes to allow the flours to absorb the liquid.
- ➤ Heat a non-stick skillet or dosa tawa over medium heat and lightly grease it with ghee or coconut oil.

- ➢ Pour a ladleful of the batter onto the center of the skillet and spread it in a circular motion to form a thin dosa.
- ➢ Cook the dosa for a couple of minutes until the edges start to turn golden brown and crisp.
- ➢ Flip the dosa and cook for another minute or so on the other side.
- ➢ Repeat the process with the remaining batter, adding more ghee or coconut oil to the skillet as needed.
- ➢ Serve the keto almond flour dosa hot with chutney, keto-friendly curry, or your preferred toppings.

Nutritional Values:

Please note that these values are approximate and may vary based on specific ingredients used and serving size.

Per serving (1 dosa):

Calories: 160
Total Fat: 14g
Saturated Fat: 2g
Total Carbohydrates: 5g (Net: 3g)
Fiber: 2g
Protein: 7g

Health Benefits:

Almond Flour: Almond flour is low in carbs and high in healthy fats, protein, and vitamin E. It may contribute to heart health and help regulate blood sugar levels.

Flaxseed Meal: Flaxseed meal is rich in omega-3 fatty acids and dietary fiber. It may promote digestive health and reduce inflammation.

How it Helps in Keto:

Keto almond flour dosa is low in net carbs and provides a good amount of healthy fats, protein, and fiber. It's a suitable alternative for those following a keto diet and looking for a grain-free option.

Best Time of the Day to Eat:

Keto almond flour dosa can be enjoyed as a savory breakfast, lunch, or dinner. It pairs well with keto-friendly chutneys, dips, or curries. Customize the fillings or toppings to suit your preferences and dietary needs.

80 Keto Baked Cheesy Zucchini

Keto baked cheesy zucchini is a flavorful and nutritious side dish or snack that highlights the natural sweetness of zucchini. It's topped with cheese and baked to perfection, creating a delicious low-carb option. Here's how you can make it:

Ingredients:

2 medium Zucchini, sliced lengthwise
2 tablespoons of Olive Oil
Salt and Pepper to taste
1/2 teaspoon of Garlic Powder
1/2 teaspoon of Dried Italian Seasoning (or your preferred herbs)
1/2 cup of Shredded Cheese (such as mozzarella, cheddar, or a blend)

Instructions:

- ➤ Preheat your oven to 200°C (400°F) and line a baking sheet with parchment paper.
- ➤ Place the sliced zucchini on the prepared baking sheet. Drizzle olive oil over the zucchini slices and season with salt, pepper, garlic powder, and dried Italian seasoning.
- ➤ Toss the zucchini gently to coat them evenly with the oil and seasonings.
- ➤ Spread the zucchini slices in a single layer on the baking sheet.
- ➤ Bake in the preheated oven for about 15-20 minutes, or until the zucchini is tender and slightly golden around the edges.

- ➢ Remove from the oven and sprinkle the shredded cheese over the zucchini slices.
- ➢ Return the baking sheet to the oven and bake for an additional 3-5 minutes, or until the cheese is melted and bubbly.
- ➢ Remove from the oven and let the baked cheesy zucchini cool slightly before serving.

Nutritional Values:

Please note that these values are approximate and may vary based on specific ingredients used and serving size.

Per serving (about 1 medium zucchini):

Calories: 180
Total Fat: 14g
Saturated Fat: 4g
Total Carbohydrates: 4g (Net: 2g)
Fiber: 2g
Protein: 10g

Health Benefits:

Zucchini: Zucchini is low in calories and carbohydrates. It's a good source of vitamins A and C, potassium, and antioxidants.
Cheese: Cheese provides protein, calcium, and other essential nutrients. It can support bone health and may contribute to satiety.

How it Helps in Keto:

Keto baked cheesy zucchini is low in net carbs and provides a moderate amount of healthy fats and protein. It's a satisfying option that can be enjoyed as a side dish or a snack.

Best Time of the Day to Eat:

Keto baked cheesy zucchini can be enjoyed as a side dish for lunch or dinner. It pairs well with grilled meats or can be served as a snack or appetizer. Customize it with your preferred cheese or additional toppings to suit your taste.

81 Keto Spiced Almond Butter

Keto spiced almond butter is a delicious and nutritious spread that can be enjoyed on its own or used as an ingredient in various recipes. It's made with roasted almonds and a blend of aromatic spices, creating a flavorful option for keto enthusiasts. Here's how you can make it:

Ingredients:

2 cups of Roasted Almonds
2 tablespoons of Coconut Oil, melted
1 tablespoon of Erythritol or your preferred keto-friendly sweetener (optional)
1 teaspoon of Ground Cinnamon
1/2 teaspoon of Ground Ginger
1/4 teaspoon of Ground Nutmeg
1/4 teaspoon of Ground Cloves
1/4 teaspoon of Salt

Instructions:

- ➢ Place the roasted almonds in a food processor or high-powered blender.
- ➢ Process the almonds for a few minutes, scraping down the sides occasionally, until they start to release their natural

oils and turn into a smooth and creamy consistency. This process may take some time, so be patient.

➢ Add the melted coconut oil, erythritol (if using), ground cinnamon, ground ginger, ground nutmeg, ground cloves, and salt to the food processor or blender.

➢ Continue processing until all the ingredients are well combined and the almond butter is smooth and creamy.

➢ Taste and adjust the sweetness or spice levels to your preference.

➢ Transfer the spiced almond butter to a clean and airtight jar.

➢ Store it in the refrigerator for up to a month or at room temperature for a week.

Nutritional Values:

Please note that these values are approximate and may vary based on specific ingredients used and serving size.

Per serving (2 tablespoons):

Calories: 190
Total Fat: 18g
Saturated Fat: 4g
Total Carbohydrates: 5g (Net: 3g)
Fiber: 2g
Protein: 5g

Health Benefits:

Almonds: Almonds are a good source of healthy fats, protein, fiber, vitamin E, and magnesium. They may support heart health and help manage blood sugar levels.

Spices: The spices used in this recipe, such as cinnamon, ginger, nutmeg, and cloves, not only add flavor but also provide potential health benefits due to their antioxidant and anti-inflammatory properties.

How it Helps in Keto:

Keto spiced almond butter is low in net carbs and provides a good amount of healthy fats, fiber, and protein. It's a convenient and tasty option for adding nutrient-dense ingredients to a keto diet.

Best Time of the Day to Eat:

Keto spiced almond butter can be enjoyed at any time of the day. Spread it on keto-friendly bread, use it as a dip for low-carb fruits or vegetables, or incorporate it into your favorite keto recipes. It's a versatile and satisfying option that can add flavor and nutrition to your meals.

82 Keto Masala Roasted Brussels Sprouts

Keto masala roasted Brussels sprouts are a flavorful and nutritious side dish that combines the earthy taste of Brussels sprouts with aromatic Indian spices. Here's how you can make it:

Ingredients:

1 pound Brussels sprouts, trimmed and halved
2 tablespoons olive oil
1 teaspoon garam masala
1/2 teaspoon ground cumin
1/2 teaspoon ground coriander
1/4 teaspoon turmeric
1/4 teaspoon chili powder (optional, for heat)
Salt to taste

Instructions:

➤ Preheat your oven to 200°C (400°F) and line a baking sheet with parchment paper.
➤ In a mixing bowl, combine the olive oil, garam masala, ground cumin, ground coriander, turmeric, chili powder (if using), and salt.
➤ Add the halved Brussels sprouts to the bowl and toss them until they are well coated with the spice mixture.
➤ Transfer the Brussels sprouts to the prepared baking sheet, spreading them out in a single layer.
➤ Roast in the preheated oven for about 20-25 minutes, or until the Brussels sprouts are tender and golden brown, stirring once or twice during cooking for even browning.

- ➢ Remove from the oven and let them cool slightly before serving.
- ➢ Nutritional Values:
- ➢ Please note that these values are approximate and may vary based on specific ingredients used and serving size.

Per serving (1/4 of the recipe):

Calories: 100
Total Fat: 7g
Saturated Fat: 1g
Total Carbohydrates: 8g (Net: 4g)
Fiber: 4g
Protein: 4g

Health Benefits:

Brussels Sprouts: Brussels sprouts are rich in vitamins C and K, fiber, and antioxidants. They may have anti-inflammatory properties and contribute to heart health.

Spices: The spices used in this recipe, such as garam masala, cumin, coriander, turmeric, and chili powder, not only add flavor but also provide potential health benefits due to their antioxidant and anti-inflammatory properties.

How it Helps in Keto:

Keto masala roasted Brussels sprouts are low in net carbs and provide a good amount of fiber and nutrients. They can be a satisfying and nutritious addition to a keto diet.

Best Time of the Day to Eat:

Keto masala roasted Brussels sprouts can be enjoyed as a side dish for lunch or dinner. They pair well with grilled meats or can be served as a snack. Incorporate them into your meal rotation to add variety and flavor.

83 Keto Paneer and Spinach Soup

Keto paneer and spinach soup is a creamy and satisfying soup that combines the richness of paneer (Indian cottage cheese) with the nutritious goodness of spinach. Here's how you can make it:

Ingredients:

2 tablespoons ghee or olive oil
1 small onion, finely chopped
2 cloves garlic, minced
1 teaspoon grated ginger
1 teaspoon cumin powder
1/2 teaspoon turmeric
1/2 teaspoon garam masala
4 cups fresh spinach leaves
1 cup paneer, cubed
4 cups vegetable broth or water
Salt and pepper to taste
Fresh cilantro for garnish (optional)

Instructions:

➤ Heat ghee or olive oil in a large pot over medium heat. Add the chopped onion and cook until translucent.
➤ Add the minced garlic and grated ginger to the pot and sauté for another minute.
➤ Stir in the cumin powder, turmeric, and garam masala, and cook for a minute until fragrant.
➤ Add the spinach leaves to the pot and cook until wilted, stirring occasionally.
➤ Remove the pot from heat and let the mixture cool slightly.

- ➢ Transfer the mixture to a blender or use an immersion blender to puree until smooth.
- ➢ Return the pureed mixture to the pot and place it back on the stove over low heat.
- ➢ Add the cubed paneer and vegetable broth or water to the pot. Stir well to combine.
- ➢ Simmer the soup for about 10-15 minutes, allowing the flavors to meld together and the paneer to soften.
- ➢ Season with salt and pepper to taste.
- ➢ Ladle the soup into bowls and garnish with fresh cilantro, if desired.

Nutritional Values:

Please note that these values are approximate and may vary based on specific ingredients used and serving size.

Per serving (1/4 of the recipe):

Calories: 220
Total Fat: 16g
Saturated Fat: 8g
Total Carbohydrates: 6g (Net: 4g)
Fiber: 2g
Protein: 14g

Health Benefits:

Paneer: Paneer is a good source of protein, calcium, and healthy fats. It can support muscle growth, bone health, and provide satiety.
Spinach: Spinach is packed with vitamins, minerals, and antioxidants. It is low in calories and carbs, and may support heart health and improve digestion.
How it Helps in Keto:

Keto paneer and spinach soup is low in net carbs and provides a good amount of healthy fats, protein, and fiber. It's a satisfying option that can be enjoyed as a meal on its own or paired with a low-carb side dish.

Best Time of the Day to Eat:

Keto paneer and spinach soup can be enjoyed for lunch or dinner. It can be a comforting and nourishing meal option, especially during colder months. Serve it with a side salad or keto-friendly bread for a complete and balanced meal.

84 Keto Roasted Tomato Soup

Keto roasted tomato soup is a comforting and flavorful soup made from roasted tomatoes and aromatic herbs. Here's how you can make it:

Ingredients:

2 pounds tomatoes, halved
2 tablespoons olive oil
1 small onion, chopped
2 cloves garlic, minced
1/2 teaspoon dried basil
1/2 teaspoon dried oregano
1/4 teaspoon dried thyme
1 cup vegetable broth
Salt and pepper to taste
Fresh basil leaves for garnish (optional)

Instructions:

➤ Preheat your oven to 200°C (400°F).
➤ Place the halved tomatoes on a baking sheet and drizzle them with olive oil. Season with salt and pepper.
➤ Roast the tomatoes in the preheated oven for about 30-40 minutes, or until they are soft and slightly caramelized.
➤ While the tomatoes are roasting, heat olive oil in a large pot over medium heat. Add the chopped onion and minced garlic. Sauté until the onion is translucent and fragrant.
➤ Add the dried basil, dried oregano, and dried thyme to the pot. Stir well to coat the onions and garlic with the herbs.
➤ Once the roasted tomatoes are ready, remove them from the oven and let them cool slightly.

- ➤ Transfer the roasted tomatoes to the pot with the onion and garlic mixture. Stir well to combine.
- ➤ Using an immersion blender or a regular blender, puree the mixture until smooth.
- ➤ Return the pot to the stove over low heat. Add the vegetable broth and simmer for about 10-15 minutes, allowing the flavors to meld together.
- ➤ Season with salt and pepper to taste.
- ➤ Ladle the soup into bowls and garnish with fresh basil leaves, if desired.

Nutritional Values:

Please note that these values are approximate and may vary based on specific ingredients used and serving size.

Per serving (1/4 of the recipe):

Calories: 90
Total Fat: 7g
Saturated Fat: 1g
Total Carbohydrates: 7g (Net: 4g)
Fiber: 3g
Protein: 2g

Health Benefits:

Tomatoes: Tomatoes are rich in vitamins A, C, and antioxidants like lycopene. They may support heart health and have anti-inflammatory properties.

Herbs: Basil, oregano, and thyme not only add flavor to the soup but also provide potential health benefits due to their antioxidant and antimicrobial properties.

How it Helps in Keto:

Keto roasted tomato soup is low in net carbs and provides a moderate amount of healthy fats and fiber. It's a comforting and nutritious option for those following a keto diet.

Best Time of the Day to Eat:

Keto roasted tomato soup can be enjoyed for lunch or dinner. It can be a comforting and satisfying meal option, especially during cooler days. Serve it with a side salad or a keto-friendly bread for a complete and balanced meal.

85 Keto Stuffed Eggplant

Keto stuffed eggplant is a delicious and filling dish that combines tender eggplant with a flavorful stuffing. Here's how you can make it:

Ingredients:

2 medium eggplants
2 tablespoons olive oil
1 small onion, chopped
2 cloves garlic, minced
1/2 cup diced bell peppers (any color)
1/2 cup diced zucchini
1/2 cup diced tomatoes
1/4 cup crumbled feta cheese
2 tablespoons chopped fresh parsley
1 teaspoon dried oregano
Salt and pepper to taste

Instructions:

➢ Preheat your oven to 200°C (400°F).
➢ Slice the eggplants in half lengthwise. Score the flesh in a crisscross pattern, being careful not to cut through the skin.
➢ Brush the cut sides of the eggplants with olive oil and place them on a baking sheet, cut side up.
➢ Bake the eggplants in the preheated oven for about 30-40 minutes, or until the flesh is tender and golden brown.
➢ While the eggplants are baking, heat olive oil in a skillet over medium heat. Add the chopped onion and minced garlic. Sauté until the onion is translucent and fragrant.

- ➢ Add the diced bell peppers, diced zucchini, and diced tomatoes to the skillet. Cook for about 5 minutes, or until the vegetables are tender.
- ➢ Remove the skillet from heat and stir in the crumbled feta cheese, chopped parsley, dried oregano, salt, and pepper.
- ➢ Once the eggplants are cooked, remove them from the oven and let them cool slightly.
- ➢ Using a spoon, gently scoop out the flesh from the eggplants, leaving a thin shell.
- ➢ Chop the scooped-out flesh and add it to the skillet with the vegetable mixture. Stir well to combine.
- ➢ Spoon the vegetable filling into the eggplant shells, pressing it down gently.
- ➢ Place the stuffed eggplants back on the baking sheet and bake for an additional 10-15 minutes, or until the filling is heated through.
- ➢ Remove from the oven and let them cool for a few minutes before serving.

Nutritional Values:

Please note that these values are approximate and may vary based on specific ingredients used and serving size.

Per serving (1/2 of the recipe):

Calories: 180
Total Fat: 10g
Saturated Fat: 2g
Total Carbohydrates: 19g (Net: 11g)
Fiber: 8g
Protein: 6g

Health Benefits:

Eggplant: Eggplants are low in calories and carbs but rich in fiber, vitamins, and minerals. They may support heart health and aid digestion.

Vegetables: Bell peppers, zucchini, and tomatoes provide an array of vitamins, minerals, and antioxidants that contribute to overall health.

How it Helps in Keto:

Keto stuffed eggplant is moderate in net carbs and provides a good amount of fiber and nutrients. It's a satisfying and flavorful option that can fit into a keto diet.

Best Time of the Day to Eat:

Keto stuffed eggplant can be enjoyed for lunch or dinner. It can be served as a main course or a side dish. Pair it with a fresh salad or a side of roasted vegetables for a complete meal.

86 Keto Grilled Eggplant with Tahini Dressing

Keto grilled eggplant with tahini dressing is a delicious and healthy dish that highlights the natural flavors of eggplant and combines it with a creamy and tangy tahini dressing. Here's how you can make it:

Ingredients:

2 medium eggplants, sliced into 1/2-inch thick rounds
2 tablespoons olive oil
Salt and pepper to taste
1/4 cup tahini
2 tablespoons lemon juice
1 clove garlic, minced
2 tablespoons chopped fresh parsley

Instructions:

- ➤ Preheat your grill to medium heat.
- ➤ Brush both sides of the eggplant slices with olive oil and season with salt and pepper.
- ➤ Grill the eggplant slices for about 4-5 minutes per side, or until they are tender and have grill marks.
- ➤ While the eggplant is grilling, prepare the tahini dressing. In a small bowl, whisk together the tahini, lemon juice, minced garlic, and a pinch of salt.
- ➤ Once the eggplant slices are cooked, remove them from the grill and let them cool slightly.
- ➤ Arrange the grilled eggplant slices on a serving platter and drizzle the tahini dressing over the top.
- ➤ Sprinkle the chopped fresh parsley on top for added freshness and flavor.

➢ Serve the grilled eggplant immediately as a side dish or as part of a larger meal.

Nutritional Values:

Please note that these values are approximate and may vary based on specific ingredients used and serving size.

Per serving (1/4 of the recipe):

Calories: 160
Total Fat: 13g
Saturated Fat: 2g
Total Carbohydrates: 9g (Net: 6g)
Fiber: 3g
Protein: 4g

Health Benefits:

Eggplant: Eggplants are low in calories and carbs but rich in fiber, vitamins, and minerals. They may support heart health and aid digestion.

Tahini: Tahini, made from ground sesame seeds, is a good source of healthy fats, protein, and minerals like calcium and iron. It may contribute to bone health and provide antioxidant benefits.

How it Helps in Keto:

Keto grilled eggplant with tahini dressing is low in net carbs and provides a moderate amount of healthy fats and fiber. It's a flavorful and satisfying option that aligns with a keto diet.

Best Time of the Day to Eat:

Keto grilled eggplant with tahini dressing can be enjoyed for lunch or dinner. It can be served as a side dish or as part of a mezze-style spread. Pair it with grilled meats or other keto-friendly vegetables for a complete meal.

87 Keto Spinach and Avocado Salad

Ingredients:

4 cups fresh spinach leaves
1 avocado, sliced
1/4 cup sliced almonds
2 tablespoons olive oil
1 tablespoon lemon juice
Salt and pepper to taste

Instructions:

➢ In a large bowl, combine the fresh spinach leaves, sliced avocado, and sliced almonds.
➢ In a small bowl, whisk together the olive oil, lemon juice, salt, and pepper to make the dressing.
➢ Pour the dressing over the salad and toss gently to coat all the ingredients.
➢ Serve the keto spinach and avocado salad immediately as a refreshing side dish or light meal.

Nutritional Values:

Please note that these values are approximate and may vary based on specific ingredients used and serving size.

Per serving (1/2 of the recipe):

Calories: 250
Total Fat: 23g
Saturated Fat: 3g
Total Carbohydrates: 9g (Net: 5g)
Fiber: 4g
Protein: 4g

Health Benefits:

Spinach: Spinach is rich in vitamins A, C, and K, as well as minerals like iron and calcium. It is low in calories and carbohydrates, and may support eye health, bone health, and immune function.

Avocado: Avocado is a good source of healthy fats, vitamins, and minerals. It may support heart health, brain function, and promote satiety.

How it Helps in Keto:

Keto spinach and avocado salad is low in net carbs and provides a good amount of healthy fats and fiber. It's a nutritious and satisfying option for those following a keto diet.

Best Time of the Day to Eat:

Keto spinach and avocado salad can be enjoyed as a light lunch or dinner. It can also be served as a side dish with grilled chicken or fish. Enjoy it whenever you crave a refreshing and nutrient-packed meal.

88 Keto Roasted Pumpkin Soup

Ingredients:

2 cups pumpkin puree (canned or homemade)
1 small onion, chopped
2 cloves garlic, minced
2 cups vegetable broth
1/2 cup heavy cream
1 teaspoon pumpkin pie spice
Salt and pepper to taste
Optional toppings: pumpkin seeds, sour cream, chopped fresh herbs

Instructions:

> Preheat your oven to 200°C (400°F).
> Place the pumpkin puree, chopped onion, and minced garlic in a large pot over medium heat. Cook for a few minutes until the onion and garlic are softened.
> Add the vegetable broth, heavy cream, pumpkin pie spice, salt, and pepper to the pot. Stir well to combine.
> Bring the mixture to a boil, then reduce the heat to low and let it simmer for about 15 minutes, allowing the flavors to meld together.
> While the soup is simmering, spread the pumpkin seeds on a baking sheet and roast them in the preheated oven for about 5-7 minutes until they are golden and crispy. Set aside.
> Remove the pot from the heat and let the soup cool slightly.
> Use an immersion blender or transfer the soup to a blender to puree until smooth.
> Return the soup to the pot and reheat it over low heat if needed.

- ➢ Ladle the keto roasted pumpkin soup into bowls and garnish with roasted pumpkin seeds, a dollop of sour cream, or chopped fresh herbs, if desired.

Nutritional Values:

Please note that these values are approximate and may vary based on specific ingredients used and serving size.

Per serving (1/4 of the recipe):

Calories: 180
Total Fat: 15g
Saturated Fat: 9g
Total Carbohydrates: 9g (Net: 7g)
Fiber: 2g
Protein: 3g

Health Benefits:

Pumpkin: Pumpkin is low in calories and carbs but rich in fiber, vitamins A, C, and potassium. It may support eye health, aid digestion, and boost immune function.

Vegetable Broth: Vegetable broth provides hydration and can contribute to your daily vegetable intake.

How it Helps in Keto:

Keto roasted pumpkin soup is moderate in net carbs and provides a good amount of healthy fats and fiber. It's a comforting and flavorful option that can be enjoyed on a keto diet.

Best Time of the Day to Eat:

Keto roasted pumpkin soup can be enjoyed for lunch or dinner. It can be served as a light meal on its own or paired with a keto-friendly salad or protein. It's particularly popular during the fall season.

89 Keto Spicy Roasted Cabbage

Ingredients:

1 small head of cabbage, cut into wedges
2 tablespoons olive oil
1 teaspoon paprika
1/2 teaspoon garlic powder
1/2 teaspoon onion powder
1/4 teaspoon cayenne pepper (adjust to taste)
Salt and pepper to taste
Fresh parsley for garnish (optional)

Instructions:

- ➢ Preheat your oven to 220°C (425°F).
- ➢ Place the cabbage wedges on a baking sheet lined with parchment paper.
- ➢ In a small bowl, combine the olive oil, paprika, garlic powder, onion powder, cayenne pepper, salt, and pepper. Stir well to make a spice mixture.
- ➢ Brush the spice mixture evenly over the cabbage wedges, making sure to coat all sides.
- ➢ Roast the cabbage in the preheated oven for about 20-25 minutes, or until the edges are crispy and golden brown.
- ➢ Remove from the oven and let the spicy roasted cabbage cool slightly.
- ➢ Garnish with fresh parsley, if desired, before serving.

Nutritional Values:

Please note that these values are approximate and may vary based on specific ingredients used and serving size.

Per serving (1/4 of the recipe):

Calories: 90
Total Fat: 7g
Saturated Fat: 1g
Total Carbohydrates: 7g (Net: 5g)
Fiber: 2g
Protein: 2g

Health Benefits:

Cabbage: Cabbage is low in calories and carbs but high in fiber, vitamins C and K, and antioxidants. It may support digestion, promote heart health, and contribute to a healthy immune system.

How it Helps in Keto:

Keto spicy roasted cabbage is low in net carbs and provides a moderate amount of healthy fats and fiber. It's a flavorful and satisfying side dish that fits well into a keto diet.

Best Time of the Day to Eat:

Keto spicy roasted cabbage can be enjoyed as a side dish for lunch or dinner. It pairs well with grilled meats or can be used as a base for a vegetarian meal. Serve it warm or at room temperature.

90 Keto Grilled Paneer Salad

Ingredients:

200g paneer, cut into cubes
2 cups mixed salad greens (such as lettuce, spinach, or arugula)
1 cucumber, sliced
1 bell pepper, sliced
1 small red onion, sliced
2 tablespoons olive oil
1 tablespoon lemon juice
1/2 teaspoon cumin powder
Salt and pepper to taste
Fresh cilantro for garnish (optional)

Instructions:

- Preheat your grill or grill pan to medium-high heat.
- In a bowl, combine the paneer cubes, olive oil, lemon juice, cumin powder, salt, and pepper. Toss to coat the paneer well.
- Grill the paneer cubes for about 2-3 minutes per side, or until they are lightly charred and heated through.
- Meanwhile, prepare the salad by arranging the mixed greens, cucumber slices, bell pepper slices, and red onion slices on a serving platter.
- Once the paneer cubes are grilled, remove them from the grill and let them cool slightly.
- Arrange the grilled paneer cubes on top of the salad.
- Garnish with fresh cilantro, if desired.
- Serve the keto grilled paneer salad immediately as a light and satisfying meal.

Nutritional Values:

Please note that these values are approximate and may vary based on specific ingredients used and serving size.

Per serving (1/2 of the recipe):

Calories: 280
Total Fat: 24g
Saturated Fat: 9g
Total Carbohydrates: 9g (Net: 6g)
Fiber: 3g
Protein: 10g

Health Benefits:

Paneer: Paneer, a type of Indian cheese made from milk, is a good source of protein and calcium. It may support bone health, aid in muscle growth and repair, and provide satiety.
Vegetables: The mixed salad greens, cucumber, bell pepper, and red onion provide an array of vitamins, minerals, and antioxidants that contribute to overall health.

How it Helps in Keto:

Keto grilled paneer salad is low in net carbs and provides a good amount of protein and healthy fats. It's a flavorful and nutritious option for those following a keto diet.

Best Time of the Day to Eat:

Keto grilled paneer salad can be enjoyed for lunch or dinner. It can be served as a main course or a side dish. Pair it with a keto-friendly dressing or a sprinkle of crushed black pepper for added flavor.

91 Keto Cucumber and Tomato Salad

Ingredients:

2 medium cucumbers, thinly sliced
2 medium tomatoes, diced
1/4 cup red onion, thinly sliced
2 tablespoons fresh lemon juice
2 tablespoons extra-virgin olive oil
1 tablespoon chopped fresh dill
Salt and pepper to taste

Instructions:

➢ In a large bowl, combine the sliced cucumbers, diced tomatoes, and sliced red onion.
➢ In a small bowl, whisk together the fresh lemon juice, extra-virgin olive oil, chopped fresh dill, salt, and pepper to make the dressing.
➢ Pour the dressing over the cucumber and tomato mixture. Toss gently to coat all the ingredients.
➢ Let the keto cucumber and tomato salad sit for about 10 minutes to allow the flavors to meld together.
➢ Serve the salad chilled as a refreshing side dish or light meal.

Nutritional Values:

Please note that these values are approximate and may vary based on specific ingredients used and serving size.

Per serving (1/2 of the recipe):

Calories: 90
Total Fat: 7g

Saturated Fat: 1g
Total Carbohydrates: 7g (Net: 4g)
Fiber: 3g
Protein: 2g

Health Benefits:

Cucumber: Cucumber is low in calories and carbs and high in water content. It provides hydration and is a good source of vitamins and minerals.

Tomato: Tomatoes are rich in vitamins A and C, as well as antioxidants like lycopene. They may support heart health and provide skin benefits.

How it Helps in Keto:

Keto cucumber and tomato salad is low in net carbs and provides hydration, fiber, and essential nutrients. It's a light and refreshing option for a keto diet.

Best Time of the Day to Eat:

Keto cucumber and tomato salad can be enjoyed as a side dish for lunch or dinner. It pairs well with grilled protein or can be served as part of a larger salad bowl. Enjoy it chilled on a hot day or when you need a light and hydrating meal option.

92 Keto Stuffed Bell Peppers with Cauliflower Rice

Ingredients:

4 bell peppers (any color)
2 cups cauliflower rice
1/2 cup diced onion
1/2 cup diced tomatoes
1/2 cup shredded cheese (such as cheddar or mozzarella)
1 tablespoon olive oil
1 teaspoon garlic powder
1 teaspoon paprika
Salt and pepper to taste
Optional toppings: fresh herbs, hot sauce

Instructions:

➤ Preheat your oven to 200°C (400°F).
➤ Cut off the tops of the bell peppers and remove the seeds and membranes.
➤ In a skillet, heat the olive oil over medium heat. Add the diced onion and sauté until translucent.
➤ Add the cauliflower rice to the skillet and cook for about 5 minutes, until it softens slightly.
➤ Stir in the diced tomatoes, garlic powder, paprika, salt, and pepper. Cook for an additional 2-3 minutes.
➤ Remove the skillet from the heat and stir in the shredded cheese until melted and well combined.
➤ Stuff the bell peppers with the cauliflower rice mixture, pressing it down gently.
➤ Place the stuffed bell peppers in a baking dish and bake in the preheated oven for about 20-25 minutes, until the peppers are tender and the cheese is melted and bubbly.

- ➢ Remove from the oven and let the stuffed bell peppers cool slightly before serving.
- ➢ Garnish with fresh herbs and drizzle with hot sauce, if desired.

Nutritional Values:

Please note that these values are approximate and may vary based on specific ingredients used and serving size.

Per serving (1 stuffed bell pepper):

Calories: 160
Total Fat: 10g
Saturated Fat: 4g
Total Carbohydrates: 11g (Net: 7g)
Fiber: 4g
Protein: 8g

Health Benefits:

Bell Peppers: Bell peppers are rich in vitamins A and C, as well as antioxidants. They may support eye health, boost the immune system, and provide anti-inflammatory benefits.

Cauliflower: Cauliflower is low in calories and carbs but high in fiber and various vitamins and minerals. It may support digestion, provide antioxidants, and contribute to overall health.

How it Helps in Keto:

Keto stuffed bell peppers with cauliflower rice are low in net carbs and provide a good amount of fiber and healthy fats. They are a flavorful and satisfying option for those following a keto diet.

Best Time of the Day to Eat:

Keto stuffed bell peppers can be enjoyed for lunch or dinner. Serve them as a main course with a side salad or additional vegetables. They can also be prepared in advance and reheated for a quick and convenient meal.

93 Keto Grilled Zucchini with Parmesan

Ingredients:

2 medium zucchini, sliced lengthwise
2 tablespoons olive oil
1 teaspoon garlic powder
1/2 teaspoon dried oregano
Salt and pepper to taste
1/4 cup grated Parmesan cheese
Fresh basil for garnish (optional)

Instructions:

➢ Preheat your grill or grill pan to medium-high heat.
➢ In a bowl, combine the olive oil, garlic powder, dried oregano, salt, and pepper.
➢ Brush both sides of the zucchini slices with the olive oil mixture.
➢ Place the zucchini slices on the grill and cook for about 2-3 minutes per side, or until they are tender and grill marks appear.
➢ Remove the zucchini from the grill and transfer to a serving platter.
➢ Sprinkle the grated Parmesan cheese over the grilled zucchini slices while they are still warm.
➢ Garnish with fresh basil, if desired, before serving.

Nutritional Values:

Please note that these values are approximate and may vary based on specific ingredients used and serving size.

Per serving (1/2 of the recipe):

Calories: 120
Total Fat: 10g
Saturated Fat: 2g
Total Carbohydrates: 4g (Net: 3g)
Fiber: 1g
Protein: 4g

Health Benefits:

Zucchini: Zucchini is low in calories and carbs and high in water content. It provides hydration and is a good source of vitamins and minerals.

Parmesan Cheese: Parmesan cheese is a good source of protein and calcium. It may support bone health and provide flavor without adding many carbs.

How it Helps in Keto:

Keto grilled zucchini with Parmesan is low in net carbs and provides a moderate amount of healthy fats and protein. It's a delicious and nutritious option for those following a keto diet.

Best Time of the Day to Eat:

Keto grilled zucchini can be enjoyed as a side dish for lunch or dinner. Serve it alongside grilled meats or as part of a larger meal. It's a great addition to summer barbecues or as a light and flavorful vegetable option.

94 Keto Avocado and Kale Smoothie

Ingredients:

1/2 ripe avocado
1 cup kale leaves, stems removed
1 cup unsweetened almond milk
1/4 cup full-fat coconut milk
1 tablespoon chia seeds
1 tablespoon almond butter
1 tablespoon lemon juice
Optional: sweetener of choice (such as stevia or erythritol) to taste

Instructions:

➢ In a blender, combine the avocado, kale leaves, almond milk, coconut milk, chia seeds, almond butter, lemon juice, and sweetener if desired.
➢ Blend until smooth and creamy, adjusting the consistency with additional almond milk if needed.
➢ Taste and add more sweetener if desired.
➢ Pour the keto avocado and kale smoothie into a glass and serve chilled.

Nutritional Values:

Please note that these values are approximate and may vary based on specific ingredients used and serving size.

Per serving (1 smoothie):

Calories: 290
Total Fat: 25g
Saturated Fat: 9g

Total Carbohydrates: 11g (Net: 5g)
Fiber: 6g
Protein: 6g

Health Benefits:

Avocado: Avocado is a good source of healthy fats, fiber, vitamins, and minerals. It may support heart health, provide satiety, and contribute to skin and eye health.

Kale: Kale is packed with nutrients, including vitamins A, C, and K, as well as antioxidants and fiber. It may support immune function, provide anti-inflammatory benefits, and support digestion.

How it Helps in Keto:

Keto avocado and kale smoothie is low in net carbs and provides a good amount of healthy fats and fiber. It's a nutritious and filling option for a keto diet.

Best Time of the Day to Eat:

Keto avocado and kale smoothie can be enjoyed as a quick and nutritious breakfast or as a snack during the day. It's a convenient way to incorporate healthy fats and greens into your keto diet.

95 Keto Cauliflower Hummus

Ingredients:

2 cups cauliflower florets
2 tablespoons tahini
2 tablespoons olive oil
2 tablespoons lemon juice
2 cloves garlic, minced
1/2 teaspoon cumin
1/4 teaspoon paprika
Salt and pepper to taste
Optional toppings: olive oil, paprika, fresh herbs

Instructions:

- ➤ Steam or boil the cauliflower florets until they are tender.
- ➤ Drain the cauliflower and let it cool slightly.
- ➤ In a food processor, combine the cooked cauliflower, tahini, olive oil, lemon juice, minced garlic, cumin, paprika, salt, and pepper.
- ➤ Process until smooth and creamy, scraping down the sides of the processor as needed.
- ➤ Taste and adjust the seasonings if needed.
- ➤ Transfer the keto cauliflower hummus to a serving bowl.
- ➤ Drizzle with olive oil, sprinkle with paprika, and garnish with fresh herbs if desired.
- ➤ Serve with keto-friendly dippers such as cucumber slices, celery sticks, or bell pepper strips.

Nutritional Values:

Please note that these values are approximate and may vary based on specific ingredients used and serving size.

Per serving (2 tablespoons):

Calories: 60
Total Fat: 6g
Saturated Fat: 1g
Total Carbohydrates: 2g (Net: 1g)
Fiber: 1g
Protein: 1g

Health Benefits:

Cauliflower: Cauliflower is low in calories and carbs but high in fiber and various vitamins and minerals. It may support digestion, provide antioxidants, and contribute to overall health. Tahini: Tahini, made from sesame seeds, is a good source of healthy fats, protein, and minerals like calcium and iron. It may support bone health and provide a nutty flavor to dishes.

How it Helps in Keto:

Keto cauliflower hummus is low in net carbs and provides a good amount of healthy fats and fiber. It's a delicious alternative to traditional chickpea-based hummus for those following a keto diet.

Best Time of the Day to Eat:

Keto cauliflower hummus can be enjoyed as a snack or appetizer at any time of the day. It's a great addition to a party platter or a quick and satisfying snack between meals.

96 Keto Tandoori Mushrooms

Ingredients:

1 pound button mushrooms
1/4 cup plain Greek yogurt
2 tablespoons lemon juice
2 tablespoons olive oil
2 cloves garlic, minced
1 tablespoon Tandoori masala spice blend
1 teaspoon paprika
1/2 teaspoon ground cumin
1/2 teaspoon ground coriander
1/4 teaspoon turmeric
Salt and pepper to taste
Fresh cilantro for garnish (optional)

Instructions:

- Preheat your oven to 200°C (400°F).
- Clean the mushrooms and remove the stems.
- In a bowl, whisk together the Greek yogurt, lemon juice, olive oil, minced garlic, Tandoori masala spice blend, paprika, ground cumin, ground coriander, turmeric, salt, and pepper.
- Add the mushrooms to the bowl and toss to coat them well with the marinade.
- Let the mushrooms marinate for about 20 minutes to allow the flavors to develop.
- Arrange the marinated mushrooms in a single layer on a baking sheet lined with parchment paper.
- Bake in the preheated oven for 15-20 minutes, or until the mushrooms are tender and lightly browned.
- Remove from the oven and let the keto Tandoori mushrooms cool slightly before serving.

➤ Garnish with fresh cilantro, if desired.

Nutritional Values:

Please note that these values are approximate and may vary based on specific ingredients used and serving size.

Per serving (1/4 of the recipe):

Calories: 90
Total Fat: 6g
Saturated Fat: 1g
Total Carbohydrates: 5g (Net: 3g)
Fiber: 2g
Protein: 4g

Health Benefits:

Mushrooms: Mushrooms are low in calories and carbs but high in essential nutrients like B vitamins, copper, and selenium. They may support immune function and provide antioxidants.
Greek Yogurt: Greek yogurt is a good source of protein, calcium, and probiotics. It may support gut health, bone health, and muscle recovery.

How it Helps in Keto:

Keto Tandoori mushrooms are low in net carbs and provide a moderate amount of protein and healthy fats. They are a flavorful and satisfying option for those following a keto diet.

Best Time of the Day to Eat:

Keto Tandoori mushrooms can be enjoyed as a side dish or appetizer for lunch or dinner. Serve them alongside grilled meat or fish or as part of a larger Indian-inspired meal. They also make a great addition to meal preps and picnics.

97 Keto Broccoli and Cheddar Soup

Ingredients:

2 cups broccoli florets
1 small onion, diced
2 cloves garlic, minced
2 cups vegetable broth
1 cup heavy cream
1 cup shredded cheddar cheese
2 tablespoons butter
Salt and pepper to taste

Instructions:

➢ In a large pot, melt the butter over medium heat.
➢ Add the diced onion and minced garlic to the pot and sauté until they are softened and fragrant.
➢ Add the broccoli florets to the pot and cook for a few minutes until they are slightly tender.
➢ Pour in the vegetable broth and bring the mixture to a boil. Reduce the heat and simmer for about 10 minutes, or until the broccoli is fully cooked.
➢ Using an immersion blender or a regular blender, puree the soup until smooth.
➢ Return the soup to the pot and stir in the heavy cream.
➢ Gradually add the shredded cheddar cheese, stirring until it is fully melted and incorporated into the soup.
➢ Season with salt and pepper to taste.
➢ Simmer the soup for a few more minutes to allow the flavors to meld together.
➢ Serve the keto broccoli and cheddar soup hot, garnished with additional shredded cheddar cheese if desired.

Nutritional Values:

Please note that these values are approximate and may vary based on specific ingredients used and serving size.

Per serving (1/4 of the recipe):

Calories: 320
Total Fat: 28g
Saturated Fat: 17g
Total Carbohydrates: 8g (Net: 6g)
Fiber: 2g
Protein: 10g

Health Benefits:

Broccoli: Broccoli is a nutrient-rich vegetable that is low in calories and carbs. It's high in fiber, vitamins A and C, and antioxidants. Broccoli may support immune function, digestion, and overall health.

Cheddar Cheese: Cheddar cheese is a good source of protein and calcium. It may support bone health and provide flavor to dishes without adding many carbs.

How it Helps in Keto:

Keto broccoli and cheddar soup is low in net carbs and provides a good amount of healthy fats and moderate protein. It's a satisfying and comforting option for those following a keto diet.

Best Time of the Day to Eat:

Keto broccoli and cheddar soup can be enjoyed as a filling lunch or dinner. Serve it with a side salad or a piece of keto-friendly bread for a complete meal. It's also a great make-ahead option for meal prep.

98 Keto Spinach and Feta Stuffed Mushrooms

Ingredients:

12 large mushrooms, stems removed
1 cup fresh spinach, chopped
1/2 cup crumbled feta cheese
1/4 cup grated Parmesan cheese
2 cloves garlic, minced
2 tablespoons olive oil
Salt and pepper to taste

Instructions:

➢ Preheat your oven to 200°C (400°F).
➢ In a skillet, heat the olive oil over medium heat.
➢ Add the minced garlic and chopped spinach to the skillet and sauté until the spinach wilts.
➢ Remove the skillet from the heat and let the mixture cool slightly.
➢ In a bowl, combine the sautéed spinach and garlic with the crumbled feta cheese and grated Parmesan cheese. Season with salt and pepper to taste.
➢ Place the mushroom caps on a baking sheet lined with parchment paper.
➢ Spoon the spinach and cheese mixture into each mushroom cap, filling it generously.
➢ Bake in the preheated oven for 15-20 minutes, or until the mushrooms are tender and the cheese is melted and lightly browned.
➢ Remove from the oven and let the stuffed mushrooms cool slightly before serving.

Nutritional Values:

Please note that these values are approximate and may vary based on specific ingredients used and serving size.

Per serving (3 stuffed mushrooms):

Calories: 180
Total Fat: 15g
Saturated Fat: 5g
Total Carbohydrates: 5g (Net: 3g)
Fiber: 2g
Protein: 8g

Health Benefits:

Spinach: Spinach is a leafy green vegetable that is low in calories and carbs but high in vitamins A, C, and K, as well as iron and antioxidants. It may support eye health, bone health, and provide various other health benefits.
Feta Cheese: Feta cheese is a tangy and flavorful cheese that is lower in fat and calories compared to some other cheeses. It's a good source of protein and calcium.

How it Helps in Keto:

Keto spinach and feta stuffed mushrooms are low in net carbs and provide a good amount of healthy fats and moderate protein. They make a delicious appetizer or side dish for those following a keto diet.

Best Time of the Day to Eat:

Keto spinach and feta stuffed mushrooms can be enjoyed as an appetizer or side dish for lunch or dinner. They also make a great addition to party platters or potlucks.

99 Keto Creamy Cauliflower Mash

Ingredients:

1 medium head cauliflower, cut into florets
2 tablespoons butter
1/4 cup heavy cream
1/4 cup grated Parmesan cheese
Salt and pepper to taste
Optional garnish: chopped fresh herbs (e.g., parsley, chives)

Instructions:

- ➤ Steam or boil the cauliflower florets until they are very tender.
- ➤ Drain the cauliflower and let it cool slightly.
- ➤ Place the cooked cauliflower in a food processor or blender.
- ➤ Add the butter, heavy cream, grated Parmesan cheese, salt, and pepper.
- ➤ Process until smooth and creamy, scraping down the sides of the processor as needed.
- ➤ Taste and adjust the seasonings if needed.
- ➤ Transfer the keto creamy cauliflower mash to a serving bowl.
- ➤ Garnish with chopped fresh herbs, if desired.
- ➤ Serve hot as a side dish alongside your favorite keto-friendly main course.

Nutritional Values:

Please note that these values are approximate and may vary based on specific ingredients used and serving size.

Per serving (1/4 of the recipe):

Calories: 130
Total Fat: 11g
Saturated Fat: 7g
Total Carbohydrates: 6g (Net: 4g)
Fiber: 2g
Protein: 4g

Health Benefits:

Cauliflower: Cauliflower is a versatile cruciferous vegetable that is low in calories and carbs but high in fiber and various vitamins and minerals. It may support digestion, provide antioxidants, and contribute to overall health.

Parmesan Cheese: Parmesan cheese is a hard cheese that adds a rich and savory flavor to dishes. It's a good source of protein and calcium.

How it Helps in Keto:

Keto creamy cauliflower mash is a satisfying and flavorful alternative to traditional mashed potatoes. It's low in net carbs and provides a good amount of healthy fats. It's a great way to enjoy a comforting side dish while following a keto diet.

Best Time of the Day to Eat:

Keto creamy cauliflower mash can be enjoyed as a side dish for lunch or dinner. It pairs well with grilled or roasted meats, poultry, or fish. It's a popular choice for holiday meals or as a comforting side during colder months.

100 Keto Spiced Roasted Pumpkin Seeds

Ingredients:

1 cup pumpkin seeds (pepitas)
1 tablespoon olive oil
1/2 teaspoon chili powder
1/2 teaspoon garlic powder
1/4 teaspoon smoked paprika
1/4 teaspoon sea salt

Instructions:

➢ Preheat your oven to 160°C (325°F).
➢ In a bowl, toss the pumpkin seeds with the olive oil until they are well coated.
➢ In a separate small bowl, combine the chili powder, garlic powder, smoked paprika, and sea salt.
➢ Sprinkle the spice mixture over the pumpkin seeds and toss until they are evenly coated.
➢ Spread the seasoned pumpkin seeds in a single layer on a baking sheet lined with parchment paper.
➢ Bake in the preheated oven for about 15-20 minutes, or until the pumpkin seeds are golden brown and crispy.
➢ Remove from the oven and let them cool completely before storing in an airtight container.

Nutritional Values:

Please note that these values are approximate and may vary based on specific ingredients used and serving size.

Per serving (1/4 cup):

Calories: 180

Total Fat: 15g
Saturated Fat: 3g
Total Carbohydrates: 4g (Net: 1g)
Fiber: 3g
Protein: 10g

Health Benefits:

Pumpkin Seeds: Pumpkin seeds are a nutritious snack that is rich in healthy fats, protein, fiber, and various vitamins and minerals. They are particularly high in magnesium, zinc, and antioxidants, which may support heart health, immunity, and overall well-being.

How it Helps in Keto:

Keto spiced roasted pumpkin seeds are a crunchy and flavorful snack option for those following a keto diet. They are low in net carbs and provide a good amount of healthy fats and protein.

Best Time of the Day to Eat:

Keto spiced roasted pumpkin seeds can be enjoyed as a snack any time of the day. They are a convenient option to have on hand for a quick and satisfying bite between meals or as a topping for salads and soups.

Motivational quotes for healthy eating

1. *"Your body is a reflection of what you eat."*

2. *"Eat well, feel well, live well."*

3. *"Health is the greatest wealth, and it starts with what you eat."*

4. *"Every bite you take is an opportunity to nourish your body."*

5. *"You are what you eat, so choose wisely."*

6. *"Don't eat less, eat right."*

7. *"A healthy outside starts from the inside."*

8. *"Eating healthy is an investment in your future."*

9. *"Good nutrition is the foundation of a healthy lifestyle."*

10. *"When you eat good, you feel good."*

11. *"Feed your body the fuel it needs to thrive."*

12. *"Healthy eating is a form of self-respect."*

13. *"Eat like you love yourself."*

14. *"You can't out-exercise a bad diet."*

15. "Eat food that serves your body, not your emotions."
16. "Nourish your body, mind, and soul with wholesome food."
17. "Make every meal a celebration of good health."
18. "Your body deserves the best, so choose nutritious food."
19. "Healthy eating is a habit, not a chore."
20. "Don't count calories, make every calorie count."
21. "Eating well is a powerful act of self-care."
22. "Treat your body like a temple, not a trash can."
23. "A healthy diet is a pathway to a vibrant life."
24. "Eating healthy is not a punishment, it's a privilege."
25. "Food is the most powerful medicine."
26. "Healthy eating is a journey, not a destination."
27. "Choose foods that make you feel alive."
28. "Eat clean, stay lean."

29. *"Strive for progress, not perfection, in your eating habits."*

30. *"Healthy eating is an act of self-love."*

31. *"Make every meal an opportunity to nourish your body."*

32. *"Food should be fuel, not a crutch."*

33. *"You don't need a miracle, just a nutritious meal."*

34. *"Eat well, be well, live well."*

35. *"Your body is a reflection of your lifestyle choices."*

36. *"Invest in your health today, or pay for it tomorrow."*

37. *"Eating healthy is a form of self-respect."*

38. *"You're one meal away from a good mood."*

39. *"Eat to nourish, not to numb."*

40. *"Healthy eating is the key to unlocking your full potential."*

41. *"Don't diet, just eat real food."*

42. *"The best project you'll ever work on is yourself, and it starts with what you eat."*

43. *"Take care of your body; it's the only place you have to live."*

44. *"A healthy diet is a solution to many problems."*

45. *"Good food choices are good investments."*

46. *"When you eat better, you feel better."*

47. *"Food is the most abused anxiety drug. Exercise is the most underutilized antidepressant."*

48. *"Don't eat less, eat smart."*

49. *"Healthy eating is a lifestyle, not a temporary fix."*

50. *"Choose health over convenience."*

51. *"Fuel your body with good food and watch it flourish."*

52. *"Your body is your temple, so treat it with respect."*

53. *"Nourish your body, mind, and soul with every meal."*

54. *"Eat like you love yourself, move like you love yourself, speak like you love yourself."*

55. *"Health is not just about what you're eating; it's also about what you're thinking and saying."*

56. *"You don't have to eat less; you just have to eat right."*

57. *"The food you eat can be either the safest and most powerful form of medicine or the slowest form of poison."*

58. *"Eat food that is grown, not made."*

59. *"Eating healthy is an act of self-discipline and self-love."*

60. *"Healthy eating is a daily commitment to yourself."*

61. *"Eat clean, train mean, live green."*

62. *"Don't dig your grave with your own knife and fork."*

63. *"When you eat good, you feel good, and when you feel good, good things happen."*

64. "Nourish your body with love and gratitude."

65. "Eat well, move well, think well."

66. "Eating healthy is not a diet; it's a lifestyle."

67. "Make food your medicine, not your poison."

68. "You can't expect to feel like a million bucks if you eat from the dollar menu."

69. "Eating healthy doesn't mean giving up your favorite foods; it means making healthier choices."

70. "Healthy eating is an investment in yourself."

71. "Don't just eat, fuel your body with purpose."

72. "Your body is your most priceless possession, so take care of it."

73. "Eat mindfully, live vibrantly."

74. "Eat food that nourishes your body and ignites your soul."

75. "You are what you eat, so don't be fast, cheap, easy, or fake."

76. "Health is not a destination; it's a way of life."

77. *"The only bad workout is the one you didn't do. The same goes for healthy eating."*

78. *"Eat like you love yourself. Move like you love yourself. Speak like you love yourself."*

79. *"Good nutrition will prevent 95% of all diseases."*

80. *"Every bite you take is an opportunity to nourish your body and transform your health."*

81. *"Eat with intention, fuel your body, and nourish your soul."*

82. *"Healthy eating is not a punishment; it's a celebration of life."*

83. *"Invest in your health today, so you can enjoy the dividends tomorrow."*

84. *"Eat clean, train dirty, live happy."*

85. *"Eating healthy isn't a sacrifice; it's an investment in yourself."*

86. *"When you eat well, you feel well, and when you feel well, you do well."*

87. *"Nourish your body, mind, and spirit with every bite."*

88. *"Eat for the body you want, not the body you have."*

89. *"Food is the most powerful tool we have to change our health."*

90. *"Health is the crown on the well person's head that only the ill person can see."*

91. *"You don't need a new diet, you need a new mindset."*

92. *"Eating healthy is a form of self-respect and self-love."*

93. *"You are one workout away from a good mood, and one healthy meal away from a great day."*

94. *"Your body is a reflection of your lifestyle, so choose wisely."*

95. *"Eat clean, stay lean, be strong."*

96. *"Healthy eating is a habit, not a chore."*

97. *"Nourish your body, and it will thank you for years to come."*

98. *"Eat food that gives you energy, not food that takes it away."*

99. *"Eat for nutrition, not just for taste."*

100. *"A healthy diet is the best cosmetic."*

Notes

Thank you

Made in the USA
Las Vegas, NV
14 June 2024

91059772R00164